Aimee Hartley

BREATHE WELL

Easy *and* effective exercises to boost energy, feel calmer, more focused *and* productive

ILLUSTRATIONS BY MIRA LOU KELLNER

Kyle Books

An Hachette UK Company
www.hachette.co.uk

First published in Great Britain in 2020 by Kyle Books, an imprint of Kyle Cathie Ltd
Carmelite House, 50 Victoria Embankment, London EC4Y 0DZ
www.kylebooks.co.uk

ISBN: 978 0 85783 802 5

Distributed in the US by Hachette Book Group, 1290 Avenue of the Americas,
4th and 5th Floors, New York, NY 10104

Distributed in Canada by Canadian Manda Group, 664 Annette St., Toronto, Ontario,
Canada M6S 2C8

Publisher: Joanna Copestick
Editor: Vicky Orchard
Editorial assistant: Sarah Kyle
Design: Emma Wells & Abby Cocovini Studio nic & lou
Illustrations: Mira Lou Kellner
Production: Lisa Pinnell

A Cataloguing in Publication record for this title is available from the British Library

Printed and bound in China

10 9 8 7 6 5 4 3 2 1

NOTE: All reasonable care has been taken in the preparation of this book, but the
information it contains is not intended to replace treatment by a qualified medical
practitioner. Before making any changes in your health regime, always consult a doctor.
While all the therapies detailed in this book are completely safe if done correctly, you
must seek professional advice if you are in any doubt about any medical condition. Any
application of the ideas and information contained in this book is at the reader's sole
discretion and risk.

CONTENTS

INTRODUCTION

You breathe, on average, around 17,000 times a day (one breath = an inhale and an exhale). If you're one of the lucky ones, and make it to the grand old age of 85, you will have around 520 million breaths to enjoy throughout your lifetime. Breathing is your very first, and will be your last, life experience. And everything in between.

For all these breaths, how does it feel to switch from the more commonly used phrase of "take a deep breath" to a new way of thinking about what it is we are doing when we breathe? What if you can learn to "make" a deep breath? And cook up a whole new way of living your life? Throughout this book I will share how, by engaging all parts of your respiratory system, you can improve the way you feel, simply by adjusting the way you breathe.

You will first bring awareness to how you breathe and learn how this influences all aspects of your life. You can then practise different breath techniques to help you feel more calm and energized. You will learn how to engage in a full diaphragmatic breath to lower your blood pressure, boost your circulation, improve your digestion and reduce feelings of stress. You can sharpen your concentration, learn the art of being present, understand how to release and heal emotions, and explore the deeper sides of your nature, all through fine-tuning and mastering your breathing.

Within these pages you will read advice, learn new breath methods, gain inspiration from respiratory consultants, world-class teachers, sleep experts, naturopaths, scientists, doctors and psychologists. As the title suggests, breathing well is the key to feeling better, and building a regular conscious breath practice, using different breath techniques, can help you to adopt an internal compass that will help you to navigate your way on the rollercoaster journey that is life.

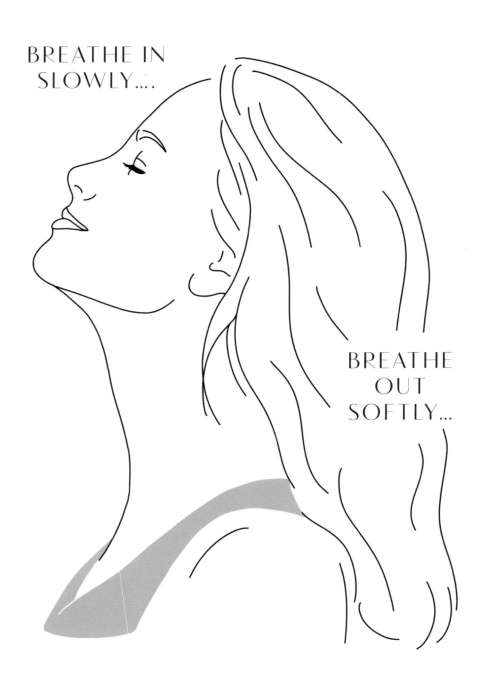

THE FOUR DIRECTIONS OF CONSCIOUS BREATHING

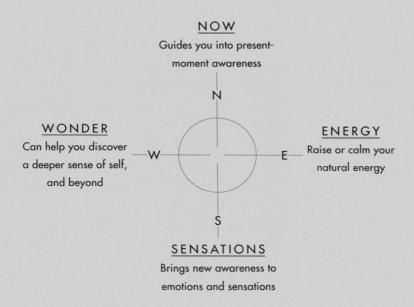

NOW
Guides you into present-moment awareness

WONDER
Can help you discover a deeper sense of self, and beyond

ENERGY
Raise or calm your natural energy

SENSATIONS
Brings new awareness to emotions and sensations

If we breathe well in all four directions of the respiratory system, pelvic and diaphragm (south), nose, throat and upper chest (north), all lobes of the left and right lungs and ribcage (east and west) we can experience the fullness of life, with a balanced state of mind.

Sometimes our first conscious breath (the one which we bring new awareness to) can be profound.

HEALTHY BELLY BREATH

When describing a full, healthy breath, I often choose the image of a toddler walking around with a big rounded belly. We can visualize the diaphragm descending fully on an inhalation, gently moving the lower organs down, which creates an unapologetic protruding of the lower belly. The entire torso moves freely with each breath and there's no muscular tension. You will never see toddlers pulling in their stomachs for photogenic purposes!

WHAT TAKES AWAY OUR "HEALTHY" BREATH?

Many aspects of our lives can impact negatively on the way we breathe. From traumatic birth experiences, unsettled family environments, the pressure to achieve the perfect figure (pulling in our bellies can trigger feelings of anxiety), to unhealthy living and working environments and the quality of the food we eat, our lifestyle can take its toll on our ability to breathe well.

I've observed the breath patterns of many children, including my own, and have noticed that we seem to lose a vital connection to our breath in the very early years of starting school. From wandering free as a toddler, breathing deeply, expressing emotions fully and living in the moment, playing and exploring without the distractions of a more mature mind, to then having to adhere to an educational regime. Sitting down for long periods, reduced playtime, along with having to deal with new social interactions and figures of authority (and the pressure of early years testing), the school environment can, for some, act as a prime catalyst for the beginnings of a dysfunctional breath pattern.

Other factors can cause our body to enter the stress response, including the quality of the air we breathe. For those living in a city, where polluted air is (tragically) the norm, I often wonder if rising stress levels are a result of us breathing less, as we subconsciously and sporadically begin to hold our breath to prevent toxins entering the body. These smaller, shallower breaths can become our default breath pattern and we can spend more of our time in an anxious "fight or flight" state. Over time this can be detrimental to our overall physical and mental health – recent research reveals that teenagers exposed to polluted air are more likely to suffer from depression.

Then there's our internal landscape, our emotions. When we don't feel able to express or engage with our feelings, our immediate reaction is to hold our breath, which prevents the natural flow of this energy and creates tension in the body. If these emotions remain unexpressed, tension can build up in the body, often within the core and respiratory muscles – and we can start to develop and sustain an inhibited breath pattern.

There are more innocent factors too – simple everyday choices like the clothes we wear can impede a full diaphragmatic breath. Tight jeans, corset-like bras, squeezed belts and restrictive fitted suits can all limit the range and depth of our breath. (Especially if worn as one outfit!)

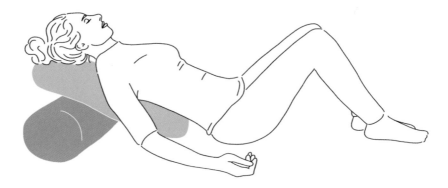

HOW DO WE LEARN TO BREATHE WELL?

The foundation of any breath practice should be re-establishing how to breathe in a full, healthy way. Subconsciously, we all know how to breathe well, we just need to spend a little more time developing a practice to remind ourselves how. This is what is should feel like:

○ Inhaling through the nose, the diaphragm descends and the belly, lower torso and lower back expand softly and fully. There should be a silent, effortless quality to the breath.

○ During the inhalation there can be an awareness of the pelvic diaphragm descending in unison with the respiratory diaphragm.

○ The ribs expand in east and west directions.

○ The upper chest and upper back lift slightly near the peak of the inhalation.

○ On exhaling, the air should exit via the nose, and the belly returns to its resting position in a calm manner.

○ The ribs will return to resting position as the lungs deflate.

○ The upper chest will also return to its rest position.

○ The rhythm of the breath should be flowing with no holding on. The inhalation should feel expansive, energizing and effortless. The exhale should be silent and smooth. A full, healthy breath should feel graceful and enlivening. The breath should support a perfect posture and vice versa.

"The wisest one-word sentence? Breathe."

TERRI GUILLEMETS

THE BENEFITS OF BREATHING WELL

The average adult breathes at a pace of around 12 breaths per minute. Each and every one of these breaths can have a positive ripple effect on all the systems of the body.

CIRCULATORY:

Slowing our breathing rate decreases stress and lowers blood pressure.

DIGESTIVE:

The diaphragm massages the stomach, intestine and colon over 10,000 times a day. Full breaths = a healthy digestive system and can improve symptoms like IBS. Diaphragmatic breathing stimulates the "rest and digest" system, which helps the nutrients in the food we eat to be absorbed more efficiently.

ENDOCRINE:

Controlled yogic breathing slows the breath rate, activating the hypothalamus, which stops stress-producing hormones (cortisol and adrenaline) from being released into the body. Consequently the body feels safe and relaxed.

INTEGUMENTARY SYSTEM (SKIN/HAIR):

Evidence shows that deep diaphragmatic breathing improves tissue functioning, and controls glucose levels, which effects the ageing of cells. Deep breaths = glowing skin.

IMMUNE:

Healthy, conscious breath holding (if you are using a full diaphragmatic breath) can increase the production of neutrophils, which are the white blood cells vital for fighting off infection and disease.

LYMPHATIC:

Seventy per cent of all toxins leave the body via the lungs, and shallow breathing can lead to lymphatic congestion. The lymphatic system relies on the muscular movement of the diaphragm to expel toxins.

MUSCULAR:

Active breath practices help strengthen and condition the muscles, by sending more oxygen, or vital energy to them. Shallow breathing can cause a lack of oxygen in the muscles and this creates physical tension in the body. A regular breath practice can release tension in the diaphragm, intercostal and core muscles, naturally allowing for a deeper, fuller and healthier breath.

NERVOUS SYSTEM:

We can move from a sympathetic to a parasympathetic state in just a few breaths. Slow, full breaths also stimulate the vagus nerve, the longest cranial nerve in the body. "Vagus" stems from the word vagabond, and this wandering nerve guides the body back into a calm and relaxed state. Research shows that an extended exhalation (if using a full diaphragmatic breath) releases a shot of vagusstoff (vagus substance) into the body, which acts like a natural tranquilizer.

REPRODUCTIVE:

A full deep breath engages the pelvic diaphragm and will increase blood flow to the ovaries and testes – which will also improve sensations during sex.

RESPIRATORY:

The only system of the body that is both voluntary and involuntary. Practising conscious breath techniques allows us to reap all the benefits of this magical system, which is the gateway to the production of energy and life itself.

SKELETAL:

A full diaphragmatic breath helps to build a healthy posture. And vice versa.

URINARY:

Deep breathing can strengthen and tone the pelvic floor, which stabilizes the function of the urinary system. Together, the respiratory and urinary systems regulate the pH of fluids.

Ultimately, a full breath will give your entire physical body much more energy!

NOSE VS MOUTH BREATHING

Breathwork has been around for 10,000 years. Yogis use it to energize the body and mind and transcend states. Athletes use it to improve their performance, midwives and doulas offer it to relieve pain during childbirth and psychologists teach mindful breath techniques to help clients retrain the nervous system. There are a plethora of techniques available for us to experience from ancient yogic pranayamas, which focus on nasal breath techniques, to the more modern open-mouth practices, such as Clarity Breathwork, Alchemy of Breath, Transformational Breath® and many more.

I love both nose and mouth breathing techniques. The more breath-controlled yogic techniques have both calming and energizing effects, while mouth-breathing techniques can help us tap into the subconscious part of ourselves, which can lead to a (temporary) esoteric state of mind.

THE NOSE KNOWS

The nose is the first port of call for the air we breathe. The nasal passageways are covered in tiny hairs or cilia and these act as a vital filtering system, clearing dust particles and irritants from the air. When we inhale through our nose, the air is warmed and humidified, making it easier for the lungs to breathe. For the health of our lungs, during everyday activities we should ALWAYS breathe through the nose.

Nitric oxide produced in the nasal cavity is an important neurotransmitter. With regular practice of nasal breathing (and conscious healthy breath-holding), we can regulate the production of nitric oxide, which can have a positive impact on our wellbeing. This "magic molecule" relays information from nerves to cells across a wide range of bodily functions, from digestion to sexual arousal. It helps to lower blood pressure by widening blood vessels and other research suggests it plays a role in memory and learning.

NASAL CYCLE

It's easy to assume that when we breathe, we use both nostrils equally. However, either your left or right nostril will be doing more of the "breathwork". Surprisingly only one nostril is working fully at any given time. This dominant nostril will switch around every 2.5 hours throughout a 24-hour period. This allows for the air filtering system in each nasal cavity to rest. Also, according to yoga texts, our dominant nostril also reveals much about our state of mind. Some nasal breath techniques (included within this book) involve a "sniff-like" action through the nose. This movement, executed well, can strengthen, tone and exercise the diaphragm creating a fuller, deeper breath.

WHICH NOSTRIL IS WORKING NOW?

O Block the left nostril and breathe in and out through the right nostril only. Take 3 or 5 breaths here.

O Now block the right nostril and breathe in and out through the left nostril only. Take 3 or 5 breaths.

O Whichever nostril is easier to breathe through is your dominant nostril!

Ancient yogis practised right nostril breathing to activate the left hemisphere of the brain and suggested if we engage in "right-nostril only" breathing, we can help activate the more creative, introspective, intuitive, artistic and poetic sides of our nature.

If you practise "left nostril only" breathing, the right side of the brain starts firing, triggering more analytical, logical and active ways of thinking. Alternate Nostril Breathing (page 165) helps the brain to find a balance between the two and has been proven to help access a more meditative state of mind.

MOUTH BREATHING

Following my years of yoga teacher training, I came across Transformational Breath® and in my first session, the certified facilitator asked me to open my mouth to breathe. The request conflicted with my yoga-trained mind so I resisted at first. An hour later I was in such a state of bliss, I felt reluctant to open my eyes and rejoin the real world.

This particular breath technique is the creation of the remarkable Dr Judith Kravitz. Judith has been teaching conscious connected breathwork for over 45 years. Here's what she has to say about the therapeutic effects of open-mouth breathing:

"Mouth breathing accesses the lower parts of the respiratory system and lower energy centres, which is where we want to begin to build our open breath — from the lower abdomen, diaphragm, then flowing upward to the chest and upper chest. I have also noticed that the seat of the subconscious is located in the lower abdominal areas, energetically and physically. So, to fully access those suppressed matters, we need to breathe fully and deeply into the lower belly and abdomen."

DR JUDITH KRAVITZ, COFOUNDER OF TRANSFORMATIONAL BREATH®

So, to breathe, or not to breathe, through the mouth? In everyday breathing, breathing in and out through the nose is sound advice to follow. For deeper, more therapeutic work, a combination of nose and mouth breath practices can be profound, and even life-changing for some.

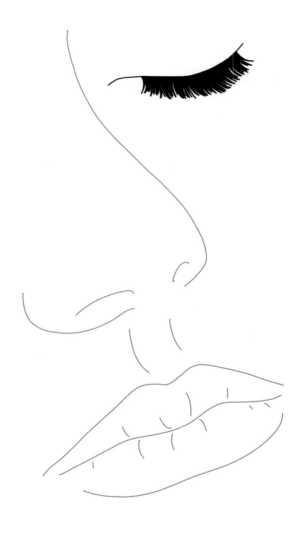

"*We don't see things as they are, we see them as we are.*"

TALMUDIC TEACHING

DISCOVER YOUR UNIQUE
BREATH PATTERN

There are around 7.6 billion people in the world and, remarkably, even though we share the same air, we all breathe in a completely unique way – the pace, rhythm and flow of our breath is as distinctive as our thumbprint.

It's helpful (and enlightening for many) to discover the characteristics of our unique breath pattern. Sometimes we need the eye of a fully trained breath worker to analyse and make sense of this pattern, helping to identify anything that might be having a negative impact on us. But luckily, we can discover much on our own.

BREATHE...

O Get as comfortable as possible. Sit or lie down, allowing the body to feel supported, either with cushions or pillows. It's important to simply observe the breath and resist the urge to consciously change the way you breathe in any way at this point.

O Gently place one hand on your lower belly (a couple of inches below the belly button) and the other on the upper chest (just below the collarbone). Take a few breaths. Where does the breath enter and leave your body? Through the nose or mouth? Simply watch where your body moves more on the inhale. The lower abdomen or upper chest? Take a few more breaths here to deepen your research.

A

IS YOUR LOWER BELLY RISING ON THE INHALATION, MORE THAN IN THE UPPER CHEST?

This can be indicative that you are a lower belly breather. This means that the diaphragm is engaged, which is a healthy foundation for the breath. Expanding the breath more into the upper chest will allow you to feel more energetic and connect more deeply with your emotions.

B

UPPER CHEST RISING MORE THAN THE BELLY ON THE INHALATION?

This can indicate that you are an upper chest breather. You may have the tendency to feel energetic, full of inspiration, but you find it hard to focus and feel grounded. Establishing a breath which is more in the lower respiratory zone (pelvic diaphragm and respiratory diaphragm) will help you to feel less anxious, more grounded and more in the present moment.

C

IS YOUR BELLY SUCKING IN AND UPPER CHEST RISING ON AN INHALATION?

This suggests you could be a reverse breather. This means everything is a bit topsy-turvy. Not to panic though, there are plenty of breath exercises within this book to help you re-establish a healthy, diaphragmatic breath. Re-engaging the pelvic floor, abdominal muscles and diaphragm to work in a healthy way can help you feel calmer, more present and less anxious.

D

BREATH IS EQUAL IN BOTH PARTS OF THE UPPER & LOWER CHEST

If you are breathing fully and there is no extensive breath-holding happening between breaths this is good news! If the breath is free flowing and fills the entire torso on the inhalation and feels expansive and effortless, and on your exhale there is a sense of ease on letting go, then you are on your way to a fuller breath. There's always room for improvement though!

BREATH TECHNIQUES
TO ESTABLISH A FULLER DIAPHRAGMATIC BREATH

Learning to breathe fully into the lower abdominal area is the first step to improving your breathing pattern. The following two techniques can strengthen and tone the primary respiratory muscles, namely the diaphragm and the deep abdominal muscles. Even if you have an established diaphragmatic breath, you will still find these techniques valuable.

TRANSFORMATIONAL BREATH®

The benefits of a Transformational Breath® practice are vast, from relieving symptoms of asthma, releasing repressed emotions and unearthing suppressed feelings of happiness and joy! It's not just the negative, more intense emotions we refuse to feel – there's so much love, happiness and joy that gets bottled-up too. Transformational Breath® is one of the most powerful breathworks I've experienced.

The foundation of this breath technique is a conscious, connected, full diaphragmatic breath. The rhythm of the breath starts in the lower belly and there should be no pauses between the inhalation and exhalation (nor between exhalation and inhalation). With a deep focus on the lower belly (and lower back), this can help you to connect with a full diaphragmatic breath. There are additional modalities involved in a guided session, such as acupressure, sound, affirmations and movement, but this short beginner's practice is safe and effective to try for a few minutes. Here's a little taster you can practise on your own.

BREATHE...

- Prop yourself up on a bed or sofa (or make a comfortable arrangement on the floor), at a semi-reclined angle so your chest is higher than your legs. Make sure you are warm and that your head and neck are properly supported. Bend the legs at the knees.

- Place your hands on your lower abdomen – a few inches below the navel. Allow the tips of the thumbs to touch and the tips of your index fingers to make a reverse triangle shape. This is your "breathing space".

- Open your mouth wide with a relaxed jaw (imagine the mouth halfway through a yawn).

- Take a long and slow inhalation through the mouth, the hands on your belly should rise with the inhalation.

- Exhale with a short, relaxed sigh.

- Keep all your focus and gentle effort on the inhalation. The inhalation should be around three times longer than the exhalation.

- The exhalation should be quiet and relaxed – a short "sigh".

- Make sure there are no pauses between the breaths.

- Repeat this conscious connected breath for 2–5 minutes.

- Notice any physical sensations in the body. Perhaps a connection with the lower belly breath? Maybe tingling in the fingers, face and toes? More energy? It's normal if your mouth feels a little dry.

- Rest for a minute as you return to a normal breathing pattern – breathing through the nose. Have a glass of water to refresh the palate.

Note: If you have a really restrictive breathing pattern and you find breathing a full diaphragmatic breath challenging, it is advisable to work with a breathing coach or Transformational Breath® facilitator.

DIAPHRAGM BREATHE

This is a nasal breath and once you have become familiar with this technique you can practise with your eyes closed. The "sniffing" action will help you exercise and strengthen your diaphragm.

O Sitting on a chair, shuffle forwards nearer to the edge of the seat.

O Place your feet hip-width apart and lean forward, so you can put your elbows on your knees and rest your chin in the palms of your hands.

O Inhale through the nose with a big "sniff-like" action, allowing the inhalation to be active, expansive and full. Breathing in, belly and lower back should expand.

O Exhale a more passive breath out through the nose.

O Notice how, in this slightly forward bending position, your belly can hang a little easier towards the thighs, allowing the diaphragm to be activated.

O Repeat for a minute. Notice how you feel. Perhaps there is more movement in the lower belly and a deeper sense of relaxation?

BREATH TECHNIQUES
TO ESTABLISH MORE BREATH IN THE UPPER CHEST

The following breath techniques are specifically for
those who have an established belly breath but inhibited
movement in the upper chest area (see pages 16–17).
(Please do NOT practise these if you are an upper chest
breather. You may feel light-headed or dizzy.)

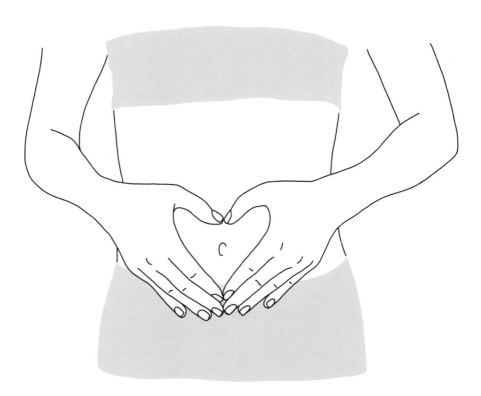

TWO-BEAT BREATHE

It's recommended to practise this with a mouth breath, but if this is uncomfortable you can breathe in and out through the nose.

○ Either sit or lie down (prop yourself up with cushions at a semi-reclined angle so your chest is higher than your legs). Make sure you are warm, and that your head and neck are properly supported.

○ Have both hands gently resting on your upper chest, just below the collar bones.

○ Open your mouth wide with a relaxed jaw (imagine the mouth halfway through a yawn) and breathe in for two strokes (two short in-breaths) so it sounds like a gentle and relaxed "ha", "ha".

○ Exhale through the mouth with a longer "haaa" sigh.

○ The rhythm should be: inhale "ha", "ha" exhale: "haaaaa". The breath should sound like a steam engine building momentum.

○ Repeat this conscious connected breath for 1–3 minutes.

○ Notice how you feel. More energized? More movement in the upper chest?

11.11.11 BREATHE

This exercise will bring your awareness and your breath into your upper chest and the breath hold at the peak of the inhalation will release a shot of the "magic molecule" nitric oxide into your system (see page 12), which will help induce feelings of relaxation. You should feel energized and calm after a minute or two of practice. If a count of 11 is too challenging, start with 6 or 7 and build up to 11 over time.

O Sit down and make sure there is length in the spine with no rigidity.

O Take your arms overhead and interlace your fingers with the palms facing upwards.

O Raise your chin without compromising your neck.

O Inhale through the nose for a count of 11.

O Hold the breath in for a count of 11. Focus on the upper chest area.

O Breathe out through the nose for a count of 11.

O Repeat for 3–5 rounds.

O Notice how the breath moves into the upper chest more naturally with the arms raised overhead.

Little and often is the key. Practising 2–5 minutes of breathwork and building up to a 20-minute daily practice will see your breath pattern improving in a short period of time. Why should we improve the way we breathe? Aren't we all surviving? Yes! But are we thriving? Possibly not.

1

WORK

"Follow your passion, and success will follow you."

TERRI GUILLEMETS

––––––––

Humans have evolved from free-moving nomadic tribes, exploring continents, plains, oceans and forests, to our largely sedentary present-day existence. In the last few generations we have started inhabiting and working in environments that require an unhealthy amount of time sitting still. From our first day at school to our last day at work, we are sitting down more than ever before, limiting our time to engage in physical activity.

This shift, from a physically demanding life – because the everyday tasks of finding food, cooking, household chores and working were far more labour-intensive – to one of relatively little movement, has occurred during a tiny fraction of human existence.

Most of us spend the majority of our lives at work, and almost 70 per cent of an office worker's time is spent sitting down. For many city dwellers being seated for 5–7 hours a day has become the norm. The modern change of pace and way of life are having a detrimental effect on our health – and on our breathing patterns. Many of us don't even leave our seats at lunchtime, so it can be beneficial for our respiratory system, our posture and our general health and wellbeing to include some form of movement and breathwork during our working day. We can use particular breath techniques to improve our posture, help free tension from the respiratory muscles and remind ourselves to move during our more sedentary days. We can enliven our workday and pep up our energy levels by practising some of the easy-to-learn breath techniques described in this chapter.

ON COMMUTE

With one in nine workers (around 3.5 million people) in the UK spending just over 20 minutes a day walking on their journey to work, a lot of us have ample opportunity to squeeze in a breath routine during our morning stroll.

The average walking commuter covers around 4km (2½ miles) to and from work (which requires around 450 breaths). With the benefits that occur from slowing your breath rate, you can easily use this valuable walking time to weave in a breath routine and arrive at your workplace, or back home, feeling calm, present and focused.

The beauty of breathwork is that you have access to it at any time of day. Our breath is like an internal health app – effective and free to use, wherever you are. Research shows that combining the right motivation (feeling better) with a 30-second action (breath exercise) and a "habit anchor" (something that you do daily) makes new routines more likely to stick.

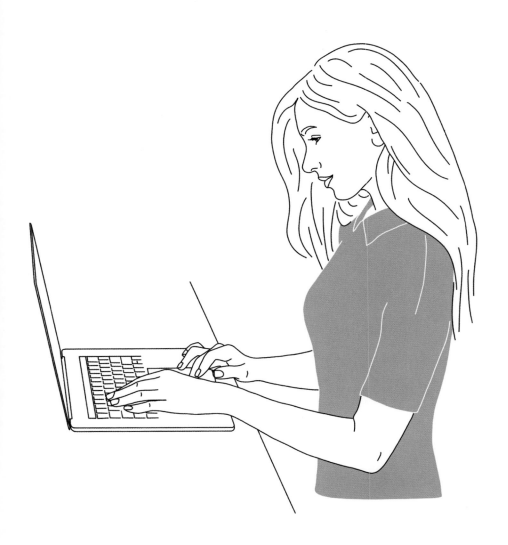

WALK + BREATHE

This simple exercise can bring you into the present moment in just one breath and one step.

When walking, bring your attention to your breathing and, when you begin to notice each breath, use this as a "metronome" to set the pace of your stroll.

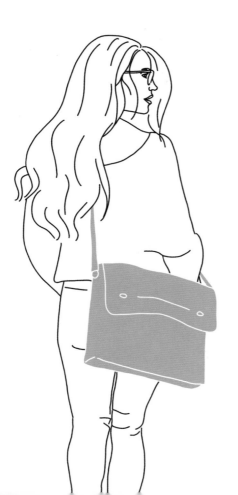

benefits

Cultivates calm

Improves focus

Lowers blood pressure

Develops a mindfulness practice – that is, an awareness of the "present moment"

Can act as a habit anchor

IT'S AS SIMPLE AS THIS:

○ Breathe in through the nose for 5 steps.

○ Breathe out through the nose for 5 steps.

○ Repeat for a few rounds and continue for as long as you can.

○ If you find the five-step count easy, then you can up the count to six or seven.

○ By slowing your breath rate to this rhythm, you may even notice that your pace of walking slows down, too. But not so much that you will be late for work!

○ Once you have found your rhythm, if your mind starts to wander, bring your attention to a part of the body with every set of steps. For instance, for five steps take your awareness to the soles of your feet. How do your feet feel today? Is your footwear too tight? Can you relax your feet a little with each step? Does the ground feel harsh on your heels?

○ With each set of steps, scan slowly upward through the body. How do your legs feel? How does the breath feel? Is it easy to breathe today? Is your breath in the belly, or is it easier to breathe from your upper chest while walking? Is your face soft and relaxed, even if you are having a bad morning? What does it feel like to smile right now? This on-the-go body scan is great for focusing the mind and slowing racing thoughts.

○ When you build up to a 5-minute daily practice, your body will enjoy all the benefits that this slower, more mindful way of breathing and walking brings.

"Our breath, like our heartbeat, is the most reliable rhythm in our lives. When we become attuned to this constant rhythm, our breath can gradually teach us to come back to the original silence of the mind."

DONNA FAHRI, YOGA TEACHER

COLOUR-LIGHT-SHAPE BREATH

Whether you travel by public transport or drive yourself, the daily commute is sometimes a catalyst for small bouts of frustration, impatience and anger (or, if you are having a lucky day, a splash of attraction). Sometimes we arrive at work having had our nervous system "ruffled", so it's advantageous to keep ourselves calm and centred en route.

You can practise this exercise while standing or sitting on public transport. (Definitely avoid it while cycling or driving, though.)

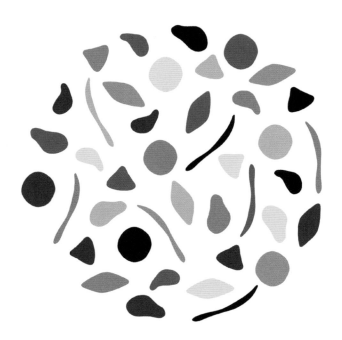

benefits

Improves circulation to the brain

Realigns posture

Releases tension in the intercostal muscles
between the ribs

Energizes the body

Calms the nerves

○ Close your eyes. Allow your spine to be tall and shoulders relaxed.

○ Take one hand to your lower belly.

○ Soften your face. Allow space between your top and bottom jaws.

○ Take in a long, slow belly breath (breathing in, the belly swells) through the nose.

○ Notice any faint colours behind your closed eyelids.

○ Exhale slowly through the nose.

○ Inhale through the nose, lengthening the in-breath a little more.

○ Notice the light and dark shades behind your eyes.

○ Exhale slowly, lengthening the out-breath through the nose.

○ Inhale slowly and calmly again through the nose.

○ Now notice the shapes you see with your eyes closed. Fix your focus on one point and notice the shapes changing.

○ Exhale through the nose.

○ Repeat for a few more breaths or until you feel calmer.

DESK DIAPHRAGM SOS
(SAVE OUR SPINES)

Your posture is the gateway to a healthy breath, and I observe many clients with a "desk diaphragm" posture, whereby the diaphragm has become so cramped under a hunched torso and an underactive ribcage that it becomes almost impossible to take a healthy breath. It's paramount, for our health and wellbeing, that we check in with our posture throughout the day, in order to help cultivate healthy breathing habits.

This is a great micro-breathing exercise for bringing energy into the upper chest and realigning the posture. It can be practised either sitting or standing.

benefits

Realigns posture

Uplifts your mood

Focuses the mind

Boosts energy

NB: If you have discovered that you are more of an "upper-chest breather" in the Unique Breath Pattern section (see pages 16–17), this exercise may make you feel a little light-headed, so stop any time you feel dizzy.

O Stand if you can; if you are deskbound, shuffle forward on your chair. Make sure your legs are uncrossed and your feet are planted on the floor, hip-width apart. If you can, always slip off your shoes, stretch your toes and plant your feet on the floor.

O Take your hands behind your back and either clasp opposite elbows or interlace your fingers behind your back, squeezing the palms of your hands and your shoulder blades gently toward each other. This movement should help lift your chest. If this is physically uncomfortable or tricky to grasp, place both hands behind your head, interlace your fingers and rest your head back in your hands. Raise the chin very slightly.

O Take 3 small breaths in through the nose. Then exhale fully with a long whisper through the mouth.

O Repeat this for a few rounds, and then you can add a breath-hold:

O Inhale 3 small breaths through the nose.

O Exhale a whispered "Haaaaaa" through the mouth.

O Hold for a count of five. Then inhale 3 short breaths through the nose.

O And exhale a whispered "Haaaaaa" through the mouth.

O Repeat for 1–2 minutes. Enjoy the energizing effects.

O Complete the exercise with a few slow shoulder shrugs: inhale through the nose, lift your shoulders to the ears, exhaling through your mouth and dropping your shoulders down.

O Repeat 5–10 times until you feel any tension release. Notice how you feel. Do you feel more alert?

ACU-CALM BREATHE "5-2-7"

This is a super-quick calmer for any stressful moments you may experience at work. It is a breath technique that can be practised undetected before a job interview, or to quell any nerves before or during a meeting, presentation or public speaking.

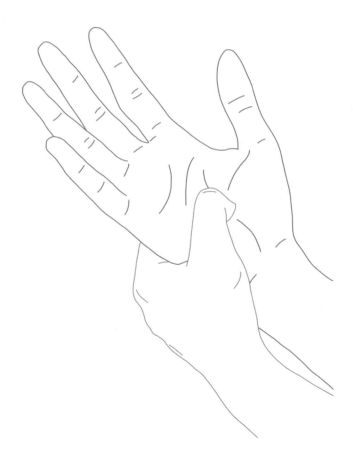

Triggers the relaxation response

Focuses the mind on the present moment

Relaxes the diaphragm

Eases stress

O Have your hands resting in your lap, with the palms facing upward. Slide your left hand under your right hand. Move your left thumb to the centre of your right palm and apply pressure. This acupressure point relates to the diaphragm and can help release tension from it.

O Close your eyes and breathe gently, with all your focus on the breath and on the pressure point in the palm of your hand. Breathe in through the nose and out through the nose or mouth, whichever feels more comfortable.

O Breathe in for a count of 5.

O Hold the breath in for a count of 2.

O Exhale for a count of 7. Repeat for 5–10 rounds.

O Repeat with your other hand.

O Notice how you are feeling. Calmer? More focused?

CHAIR NECESSITIES

I suggest to many of my clients that they take a break, or at least move little and often throughout the day, or even switch to work at a standing desk. Sitting down for 5 hours or longer has been associated with higher risks of obesity and type 2 diabetes, so we should all be taking regular walkabouts during our working day. However, if a break really isn't possible, here's a breath technique that you can enjoy from your seat.

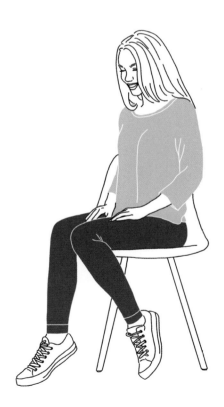

- Uncross your legs and have your feet firmly planted on the ground. Your ankles should be directly under your knees, and your legs hip-width apart. Before you start, move your legs: shake them, move your feet up and down, have a stationary jog on the spot.

- Now shuffle forward a little on your chair, so that your buttocks are resting nearer the front of the seat.

- Allow your spine to be tall and without rigidity.

- Take your arms behind you and, with your hands, clasp the lower edge of the back of the chair.

- Draw your shoulder blades toward each other gently and notice a slight lift in the upper chest.

- Gently tilt your pelvis and hips forward, allowing your belly to round toward your thighs.

- Raise your chin slightly and soften the face.

- Apply equal resistance between pulling the back of the chair toward you and squeezing your shoulder blades toward each other.

- Now that you are in position, begin to bring your awareness to the breath. Breathe in through the nose, press the tip of your tongue on the hard palate of the mouth and draw your shoulder blades further toward the centre of the spine. Imagine them nearly touching each other.

- Take in a little more air at the peak of the inhalation. There's always more.

- Breathe out through the nose and, when you feel that you have expelled all the air, push a little more out through the nose.

- Repeat for 5–10 rounds. Bring a count in here to focus the mind. Inhale "one". Exhale "two". Inhale "three". Exhale "four".

- If you need more of a stretch, bring your arms overhead, interlacing your fingers and turning your palms to the ceiling, giving the hands and fingers a good stretch and allowing the breath to flow more in the upper chest.

BOX-BREATHE

This is a well-known exercise used by the United States Navy SEALs (Sea, Air and Land teams) for dealing with stressful situations and helping them improve their ability to focus during intense situations. Regular daily practice of this can help you start your day in a calm and centred way.

---

benefits

Improves focus

Calms the mind

Brings you into the present moment

- Visualize a box as you breathe in through the nose for a slow count of 4.

- Then hold the air in the lungs for a count of 4.

- Breathe out through the nose for a slow count of 4.

- Hold the air in the lungs for a count of 4.

- Repeat for 2–5 minutes.

inhale

Visualizing the box-breathe

hold

plan

Are you feeling calmer?
More focused?

For some people, this will take just a
few rounds. If you find this count ratio
really easy, you can increase the count to
5...5...5...5; or, if you find it a challenge,
reduce it to 3...3...3...3.

exhale

BRIDGE-BREATHE

Do you arrive home still "hyped up", or exhausted, from your working day? Do you head to the fridge for a snack the minute you walk through the door, or find it difficult to unwind without the help of a glass or two of wine?

We sometimes bring our work lives home with us, and often it can be a real challenge to shake off the stresses of the day. Either of the following exercises should help you bridge the transition from work to home, after just a few minutes of practice. If you have time, always have a cold shower (see page 140) the minute you get in, too. This will help you wash away any stresses of the day.

benefits

Rebalances the nervous system

Quietens the mind

○ If you are blessed with access to a quiet room, so much the better: lie down on a bed, a couch or the floor (alternatively, this exercise can be practised in a sitting position).

○ Place one hand on your lower belly (just below the navel) and one hand on your upper chest.

○ Breathe in through the nose for a slow count of 5, encouraging the belly to expand.

○ Breathe out through the mouth, making the sound "Haaaaaa", until you reach the end of the exhalation.

○ Breathe in through the nose for a count of 5, lengthening the inhale now to bring all the breath into your upper chest, keeping your focus on the area of your heart.

○ Breathe out, closing the lips, but allowing the jaw to be relaxed. Make a soft humming sound, "Mmmmmmm", using the full length of the breath. This should feel relaxed with no strain on the vocal cords or respiratory system.

○ Repeat for 5 cycles.

○ Notice how you feel. Calmer? More peaceful?

SHAKE IT OFF

Before you engage in any household chores after work, take a couple of minutes to enjoy this practice. Sometimes all we need to do is literally "shake off the day". If you have the space, time and understanding housemates and neighbours...then dance!

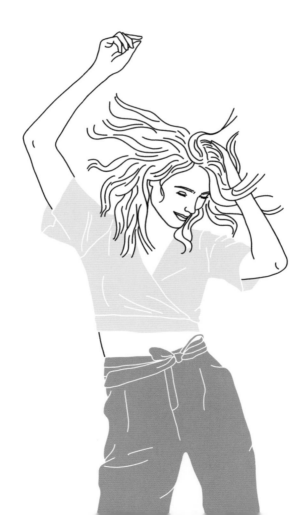

b e n e f i t s

Good for the heart

Cultivates feelings of joy

Releases tension in the body

○ Find your favourite upbeat tune, play it loudly and move your body. Become aware of how you breathe when you dance or move.

○ If dancing makes you feel a bit awkward, start by gently moving and shaking the body, beginning with the feet, ankles, legs, torso, shoulders, arms and head. Feel yourself "shake off" the day. You will feel so much lighter after doing this!

○ Continue for 3–4 minutes.

○ Then, lying down or sitting in a comfortable position, close your eyes and take 5 deep belly breaths through the nose.

○ Notice any sensations in your body. More energy in the torso? Are you feeling lighter or happier?

○ Try to think of at least two good things that happened today.

"We should consider every day lost on which we have not danced at least once."

FRIEDRICH NIETZSCHE, GERMAN PHILOSOPHER

2

TECH

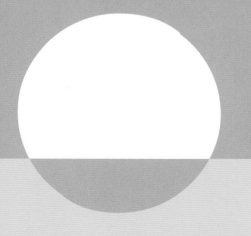

"The digital world is not home to the human spirit."

MAX STROM, BREATHING TEACHER AND AUTHOR

For some people, the digital world is a miraculous lifeline and a portal into another world, where we can learn about different cultures, study new languages and skills, talk and connect with people in faraway places and, in the same breath, buy shoes, sell houses, create businesses and even program a device for your cat to be fed while you are away – all this from a block of metal held in the palm of your hand. The mobile phone is so addictive, it's up there with nicotine (if slightly more informative and fun than a quick puff) and has almost the entire population of the West hooked.

In 2014, James Roberts, marketing professor at Baylor University in Waco, Texas, conducted a study ("The invisible addiction: Cell-phone activities and addiction among make and female college students") into the habits of smartphone users and found that mobile phone users show the same symptoms as a drug addict. He explains: "Certain people use smartphones to lift their moods. And it may take more and more time on those phones to provide the same level of enjoyment. For such people, losing a phone or having its battery die could cause anxiety or panic. That's withdrawal."

The average person will spend nearly two hours on social media every day, which translates to a total of five years and four months over a lifetime – that's a whopping 31 million breaths that we choose to use scrolling through social media.

Many of us would agree with the world-renowned breathing teacher Max Strom: that any contact with technology rarely lifts the spirit or makes the soul feel at home. In fact, there is a growing body of evidence that the more we connect with technology, the more anxious and depressed we feel. Our obsession with all things technical is at the cost of the planet's vital resources, as well as our mental health and wellbeing.

With new technological upgrades being introduced every few months, and the pressure for online "influencers" to advertise their entire life on the hour, 365 days a year, our innate messaging system can be disrupted, too. When we hear a message come through, a social-media alert or [insert shocked emoji face here] our phone actually rings, our nervous system can launch into "fight or flight" mode, mistakenly thinking we are under a real threat. Our nervous system is still primed for living in a less distracting world, and the emotional part of our brain is experiencing new feelings as a direct result of the technology boom. Even more alarming research shows that the heaviest smartphone users click, tap, type or swipe on their phone 5,427 times a day.

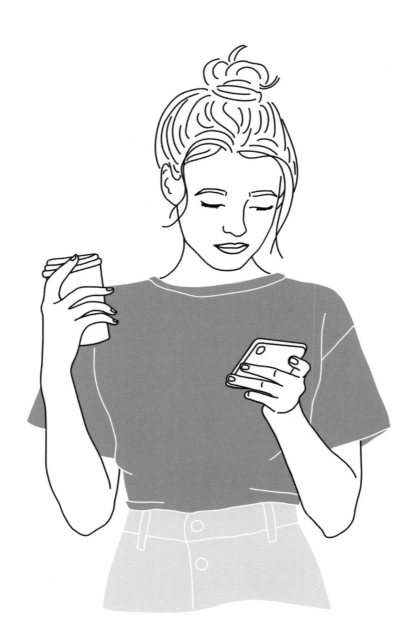

The stresses of
modern life

The latest discoveries of Dr Tiffany Watt Smith,
author of *The Book of Human Emotions*, are
rather modern emotions that I'm sure we can
all recognize:

TECHNOSTRESS
When electronic devices arouse rancorous
and stressful reactions.

CYBERCHONDRIA
Anxiety about the symptoms of an illness,
fuelled by Internet research.

RINGXIETY
According to psychologist Dr David Laramie,
who coined this term, "ringxiety" is a feeling of
low-level anxiety that causes us to think we've
heard our phones ring, even when they haven't.

That represents the top 10 per cent of phone users, so you would expect it to be excessive. However, the rest of us, on average, still have some form of touch contact with our phones more than 2,600 times a day.

This modern-day addictive behaviour draws us away from the present moment and is often so distracting that we can actually forget to breathe properly.

TECH APNOEA

A few years ago I began to notice how I held my breath while using my phone. Curious to know whether other people were doing this too, I asked many friends and clients to observe their breathing habits while using technology. I soon learned that there was a modern-day breath-holding epidemic, so I coined the phrase "tech apnoea".

WHAT HAPPENS WHEN WE HOLD OUR BREATH?

Conscious breath-holding during professionally led breathing exercises can be very beneficial to the body – so much so that it can increase your physiological and psychological endurance. The conscious breath-hold is also a production hub for the "magic molecule" nitric oxide (see the Magic-Molecule Breath on page 59), which can increase blood flow and help us to feel relaxed.

However, consistent unintentional breath-holding can cause the brain to believe that it's on standby to deal with a real threat – causing us to feel unnecessarily anxious and stressed. So the next time you are texting, scrolling, emailing, Instagramming or tweeting, start to notice how you are breathing.

"Technology is a useful servant but a dangerous master."
CHRISTIAN LOUS LANGE, NORWEGIAN POLITICAL SCIENTIST

TELLTALE SIGNS OF TECH APNOEA

Are you clenching your teeth? A tight jaw can be the first sign that the breath is being held. How is your posture: are your shoulders hunched?

A scrunched posture – chin to chest, collapsed diaphragm – will impede a full, healthy breath.

Is your breath shallow or deep?

Are you holding your breath?

BREATH-BYTES

If there is wise Buddha-like voice deep inside you,
suggesting that you need to cut back on the love affair
with your phone, laptop, TV or all things tech, then here
are a few breathing techniques that will help you to realign
your posture, deepen your breath, draw you back into the
present moment and recoup some of your real life.

The following tried-and-tested daily "breath-bytes"
will encourage you to connect with your breath before
you connect with your tech. If you can weave a healthy,
conscious breathwork routine into your life, then you will
soon reap all the benefits this can bring, including better
posture and a calmer, more present state of mind. Over
time and with practice, you will spend much more time
recharging yourself than recharging your phone.

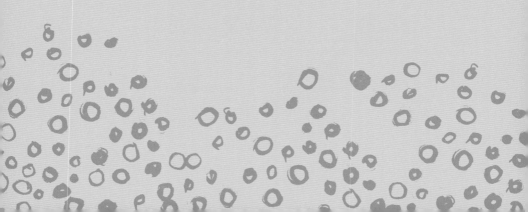

I BREATHE

Always start your day by checking in with yourself,
before checking in with your phone. This is a simple
breath-awareness exercise and, to add a bit of flavour,
you can set an intention for your day. For example, on
inhaling you can say in your mind, "I breathe in new
energy" or "I will spend less time on my phone"; and, on
exhaling, "I let go of any anxiety/stress/my hangover".

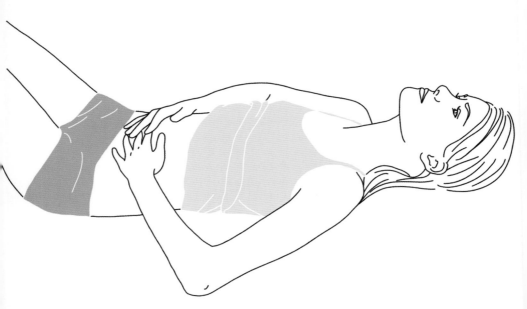

Helps you start the day in a peaceful frame of mind

Calms the nervous system

Brings you into the present moment

○ On waking, keeping your eyes closed, place both hands on your lower belly (just below the navel) and notice if it expands on the inhalation. Slow your breath down. Breathing in through the nose, slightly lengthen the inhalation, focusing your awareness on your pubic bone and your sitting bones.

○ You can visualize your breath as a wave, with your belly rising on an inhalation and falling on an exhalation. No effort or counting is needed – simply awareness. Allow your breath to enter and exit through the nose.

○ Repeat 5 more full breaths, encouraging your belly to rise a little more with each extended inhalation.

Your exhalations should be soft and quiet, and of equal length.

○ Now take your awareness to your back of your body: the space around your lumbar spine (the lowest part of the spine).

○ Take 5 breaths here, bringing your awareness to the back of your body on each inhalation and exhalation. How does your body move? Does each inhalation expand the back of your body? Does your lumbar spine descend into the mattress during an in-breath?

○ You have now taken 10 deep, slow, conscious breaths and are ready to start your day.

TECH NECK-RELIEVER

Look around any busy city and you will see a vast number
of people with their chins on their chests, gazing down at
their phones. This modern "phone pose" puts an unhealthy
strain on the back of the neck muscles (the splenius capitis,
the rhomboids, the sternocleidomastoid) and weakens the
scalene muscles (those connecting the chin and the neck).
With the majority of us being distracted by all forms of
technology for up to 5 hours a day (that's an astounding
4,000 breaths), it can be surprisingly easy to forget to take
a full, healthy breath. A lack of oxygen delivery to these
muscles results in knots, and in tension being stored within
these supporting respiratory muscles, so all forms of tech –
for all their greatness – can literally be a "pain in the neck".
Practise this exercise before and after using your phone.

benefits

Releases tension in the neck

Promotes a nasal breath

Strengthens the scalene muscles

Improves the facial muscles

NB: If you have any neck issues, you can interlace your fingers and take your hands behind the back of your head to support it in the palms of your hands – imagine your head resting in your very own hand-made hammock.

○ Whether you are standing or sitting, make sure your feet are planted evenly on the floor.

○ Take your time; tilt your chin upward enough so that you feel a stretch in the front of the throat (these muscles tend to sag when you have your chin to your chest, in "phone pose").

○ Take the tip of your tongue to the roof of your mouth and find the hard palate. Then slide the tip of the tongue back a little further and you will find a softer palate on the roof of the mouth. Apply enough pressure, with the tip of the tongue to the roof, for you to feel a lift in the front of the throat (place your fingertips on the front of the throat, just below the chin, and you should feel a slight movement here as you move the tip of the tongue backward from the hard roof to the softer palate). The movement you feel at the front of your throat is your hyoid bone (or tongue bone) – the only bone not attached to another one.

○ If you find it tricky to connect with a belly breath and the finer movements of the neck muscles, place one hand on your lower belly and lightly place the fingertips of your other hand just below the chin. Pulsate your tongue on the roof of the mouth and notice the muscles below the chin/front of the throat move. This will enable you to feel the entire landscape of your respiratory system moving outward with each in-breath.

○ Keep your head tilted backward, chin upward. Take a full, slow and lengthy inhale through the nose, and apply gentle pressure with your tongue to the hard roof of your mouth.

○ Release the pressure of your tongue as you exhale slowly through the nose. Repeat for 3–5 full breaths.

○ You can practise this again, taking the tip of your tongue to the soft palate of the roof of the mouth.

RECHARGE BREATH

This practice is often used at the end of a yoga class, to bring yogis gently out of Savasana, or relaxation. It is an effective way to bring your mind back into the present moment at any time of day, especially before and during long spells at the computer. It will also warm up your hands and give the fingertips a break.

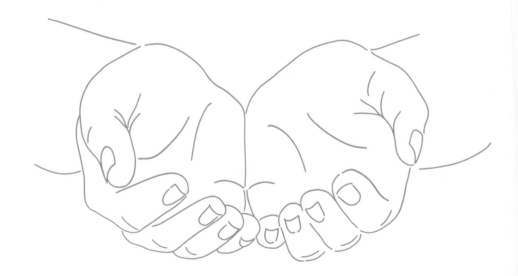

benefits

Brings you into the present moment

Boosts circulation to the hands and arms

Improves focus

O Bring your palms together and rub them vigorously up and down until you start to feel heat between them. Keep creating friction between your hands while you take 5 conscious belly breaths in and out through the nose.

O Once your hands feel quite tingly and hot, separate them, allowing a little space between them. You can imagine that you are holding an imaginary ball. You may notice the heart beating a little faster during this exercise.

O Feel the heat or vibrations anywhere in your left hand – the palm, fingertips or entire hand.

O Now take your awareness to your right hand. Do you sense any heat, vibrations or feelings here? Close your eyes to heighten the sensation. Notice any energy in between your hands. Your awareness will improve with practice, so that eventually you will be able to feel a "ball" of energy between your hands.

O Take 5 more breaths, with your hands holding this ball of energy.

O Now take your hands to your shoulders or another part of your body that you feel needs more energy.

MAGIC-MOLECULE BREATH

This is a great exercise to practise at your desk. It will keep your hands busy and help you resist the urge to pick up your phone.

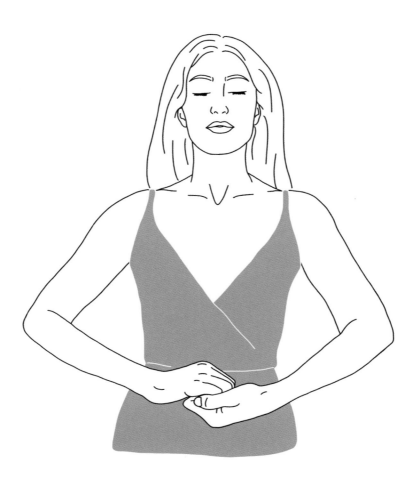

benefits

Helps boost the production of nitric oxide (see page 12)

The grip of your fingers can help strengthen your hands

Cultivates concentration and focus

○ Sitting with a tall spine, bring your hands together on your lap, with the left palm facing upward and the right palm facing down, on top of the left hand.

○ Now lock the fingertips of your left hand into the grip of your right hand, as shown.

○ Bring the sides of your hands to the lower belly, just below the navel, so that the thumb of one hand and the little finger of the other hand are close to the navel.

○ Inhale completely, and gently guide the belly into the hands. As the breath enters the lungs, increase the grip of your hands.

○ Hold the breath for 5–7 seconds (or for as long as is comfortable).

○ Exhale slowly, making sure the belly falls, and gently push your hands in toward the belly. Breathe out fully, then hold the breath for 5–7 seconds at the peak of the exhalation.

○ Repeat for 2 minutes. Switch the grip of your hands and repeat.

NB: If you have been advised to refrain from holding your breath, then enjoy this exercise simply breathing in for a count of 5, then breathing out for a count of 5.

BEE BREATH

It's good to give our eyes and ears a rest after a day in
front of the screen. Before you go to bed at night, try this
popular yogic Pranayama (breath control), which can help
calm your mind and bring relief to your eyes. First, practise
it with your eyes open, enabling you to familiarize yourself
with the instructions. Then, when you are confident with
the technique, close your eyes to enhance the experience.
The humming vibrations will boost feelings of calm.

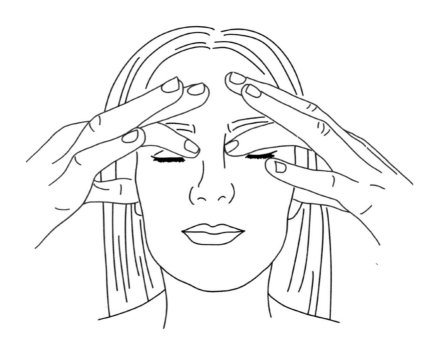

Activates the parasympathetic nervous system

Focuses the mind

Quietens negative thinking

○ Raise your hands to your face and keep your elbows level with your shoulders. Use your thumbs to close the tragus of both ears (the little flap at the entrance to your ear) and place the middle and index fingers gently over your closed eyelids.

○ Bring the tips of your little fingers under the nostrils, to track the breath entering and leaving the nose. Tune in to the inner sounds of your body. Can you hear your heart beating? Notice all the frequencies of your internal landscape. Apply a little more pressure with your thumbs if you notice any of these murmurings.

○ Take a few rounds of slow breathing here.

○ Breathe in for a count of 5.

○ Keep the mouth closed, with space between the top and bottom teeth (the jaw is relaxed) as you exhale, make a "Mmmmmmm" sound until the breath runs out. Feel the vibrations in the nasal cavity, throat and head.

○ Repeat for 5–10 rounds, noticing any sensations. If you are a well-practised yogi, then you can enjoy the Ujjayi breath on the inhalation.

NB: This exercise should never be practised with breath-holds.

Phone-fasting

The best way to avoid the "tech apnoea" trap is to reduce your use of disruptive technology altogether. Can you build any healthy habits into your daily routine? Try the following top tips to reduce your screen time.

-#NOPHONEFRIDAY

This may sound like a high-risk scenario, but try leaving your phone at home one day a week. It can be extremely liberating, and once you have got over the initial feeling that you are missing a vital organ, you will start to notice more of your surroundings. If you work from home, turn your phone to "Do not disturb" mode or turn off notifications for the entire day. It's bliss!

BUY A QUIET ALARM CLOCK

The bedroom should be a sanctuary for sleep. Banning your phone from the bedroom is one sure way to prise you from the seductive powers of the screen. If you are not soothed into a deep slumber by the sound of a ticking clock, there are quiet alarm clocks on the market, which will allow the most sensitive of sleepers to doze off and to wake in a gentle manner. The quiet alarm will emit light or vibrations that will gently alert you to open your eyes and start the day.

MINI PHONE-FAST (DON'T CHECK IN BEFORE MIDDAY)

Put your phone down at 6pm and resist the temptation to log in again before midday the following day. A "phone-fast" will help you have a better night's sleep, thereby improving your concentration and focus the next day.

"NO COMMENT"

Have a week of not "posting", "commenting" or "liking" anything. The real world will keep turning.

DIGITAL DETOX #NoWifiNoCry

Once a week (or start with just a few hours) turn off the Wi-Fi in your home. Give the house a bit of a digital detox and spend time engaged in other activities – painting, drawing or reading will have a much healthier effect on your nervous system. If you are feeling adventurous, you could spend some time off-grid – try a re-wilding weekend, where you can learn bushcraft skills, animal tracking and revisit the tasks our ancestors enjoyed, such as whittling spoons, foraging and woodcarving. And, most importantly, reconnect with nature.

CONTACT PEOPLE IN DIFFERENT WAYS

Arrange to see people in real life. This may seem to take extra effort, but is all the more worthwhile for the quality laughs and chats that last longer than 50 characters. If travelling to meet someone is a problem, buy a postcard (from a real shop!) and scribble a few words to a friend or relative.

DELETE THOSE APPS

Delete any apps that are distracting, or an obvious time-waster. This is quick and easy to do and will give you back a little bit of real time.

UN-FOLLOW THOSE ENERGY-ZAPPERS

Follow the rule "Never compare, never despair", and un-follow anyone who may give rise to feelings of inadequacy. They do not deserve your attention.

PUT YOUR PHONE IN A DIFFERENT ROOM

Resist the urge to reply to every message immediately. Create the habit of leaving your phone in a different room to where you spend the majority of your time.

REAL LIFE IS OUT THERE!

Learn to be distracted by other things: perhaps go to an art gallery or a museum, visit a place you haven't been to before or go for a country stroll, resisting the urge to take a picture or record videos. Allow yourself time to stop and smell the roses.

3

SOCIAL ANXIETY

"You may not control all the events that happen to you, but you can decide not to be reduced by them."

MAYA ANGELOU, AMERICAN POET AND MEMOIRIST

―――――――――

Social anxiety, the fear of interactions with other people in social situations, is one of the most common forms of anxiety today.

Sometimes the most exciting invitations – to a summer party, a friend's wedding or a fun work event – can act as a catalyst for unexpected waves of worry, fear and dread. We suddenly find ourselves plotting ways to politely turn down these invitations, in an attempt to evade scenarios where we find ourselves talking too much or too little, avoiding eye contact and conversations with people.

If our plot fails and we are forced to face these scenarios, we may sometimes find ourselves turning to a few extra drinks or cigarettes, to help us through. More often than not, it isn't the actual event that we want to avoid, but the feelings that may arise within us when we are exposed to these social interactions.

For some people, particular social situations can make them feel so stressed and anxious that jittery feelings start to arise, even before arriving at the event. Their breath rate can increase, as they over-worry about walking into a crowded room alone; their heart can race, with the dread of not knowing anyone; or, when faced with the challenge of public speaking, for example, they may find that their anxiety is so acute that they begin to perspire or shake.

All these feelings are indicators that the nervous system is under pressure and is in a sympathetic state, which activates the fight or flight response. Dealing with such intense anxiety can sometimes make us feel uncomfortable and slightly out of control. Luckily, if we are forearmed with a few selfcalming techniques, these unwelcome feelings can be dissipated with just a few conscious breaths.

Everyone feels anxious at certain points in their life – it is almost unavoidable. Knowing and practising healthy ways to manage our response to these uneasy feelings can play a positive role in helping us to enjoy, rather than avoid, social situations. Overcoming social anxiety can also help us cultivate confidence and resilience – and so sometimes a little stress can be good for us. There are some super-quick calmers, such as Acu-Calm Breathe "5–2–7" (see page 35) and Box Breathe (see pages 38–39), which will help to quash any nerves, but if you have a little more time to prepare, then read on for some tried-and tested relaxing breathing exercises to take the edge off any testing social situations.

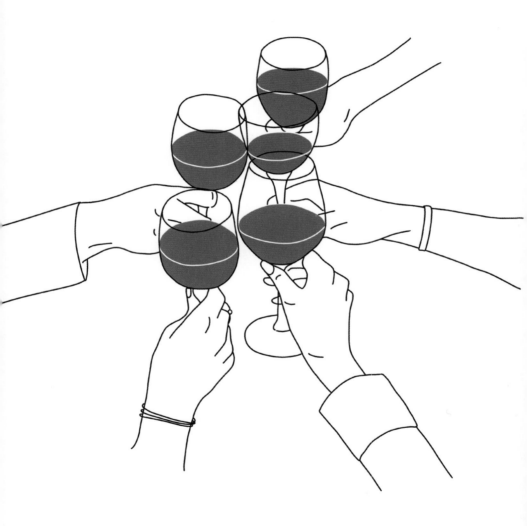

BREATHE WITH ESSENTIAL OILS

Your sense of smell is 10,000 times more sensitive than your sense of taste, and the nerves involved in smelling are closely linked to the autonomic nervous system and the emotional centre of your brain.

Inhaling specific essential oils while practising a simple diaphragmatic breathing technique can enhance its beneficial effects (see below).

Choose an essential oil that you like and mix a few drops with a base oil, such as coconut or almond. Some suggestions that are proven to help with anxiety are:

○ Wild orange or jasmine – great for confidence and energy; perfect if you have a job interview or are feeling nervous before a date.

○ Rose or bergamot – best for reducing your heart rate and blood pressure; especially effective before public speaking, to calm the nerves.

○ Lavender – effective for finding calm; the perfect antidote to any form of social anxiety.

Apply your chosen essential oil to any of your pulse points: behind your ears, at the base of your neck, on your wrist creases, inside your elbows or behind your knees. If you are on the move, you can also apply a few drops to a tissue and inhale the essential oil directly.

benefits

Bringing the breath rate down to six breaths a minute (by breathing in for five seconds, then out for five seconds) activates the parasympathetic nervous system.

The positive effects of the essential oil can help your mind and body enter a state of calm.

O Sit comfortably, close your eyes and slowly start to scan your body from your feet up to the top of your head, bringing your awareness to any areas of tension. Scan the left side of your body, then the right side. Is one side feeling lighter than the other?

O Where any tension is present, envisage a small balloon in this area of your body and focus on bringing the breath to it.

O Breathe in (through the nose) and visualize the balloon inflating to the count of 5, have a sense of creating space in this area of your body.

O Breathe out (through the mouth with pursed lips, as if breathing out through a straw) for a count of 5.

O Repeat 6 times or more until the tension dissipates, then move on to see if you can find another tense area of your body that you can breathe into.

"Sometimes the most important thing in a whole day is the rest we take between two deep breaths."

ETTY HILLESUM, DUTCH DIARIST

SELF-ACUPRESSURE BREATHE

Sometimes an extreme level of anxiety can turn into a panic attack and you may experience chest pain, heart palpitations and extreme difficulty in breathing. Panic attacks and the anxiety that causes them can actually relate to an emotional imbalance. Applying acupressure (light touch) to certain areas of the body can relieve anxiety and balance the emotions by releasing muscular tension; and it can easily be self-administered. With the tension released, your breathing will naturally deepen and you will automatically feel calmer – perfect for getting your anxiety under control and resetting the nervous system.

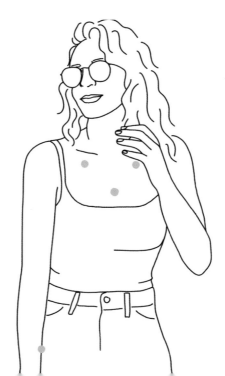

- When you are feeling anxious or nervous, there is one acupressure point that is by far the best for relief. This lies at the centre of your breastbone and is easy to find – it is four finger-widths up from the base of your breastbone/sternum. Find the n-shaped groove where the ribs meet at the front of the body. Place your little finger on the groove and measure four finger-widths up from here. Now press this point with either one or two fingers and really focus on taking slow, long and smooth breaths into this point for a few minutes. This can release tension in your chest and should leave you feeling calmer and more centred. You can add a very slow and mindful count to this, too – so inhale 1...exhale 2...inhale 3...exhale...4 – until you reach 10 or 20. Make sure you are counting very slowly, to help calm the breath down and refocus the mind.

- If you feel a panic attack looming, you can regain control using all your fingertips to press on points just below the collarbones, on the upper chest area. Press on the points on the inner side of where your shoulder meets your collarbone, and then three finger-widths directly below, as shown. Find a tender spot in this area and keep your fingers pressed there. Again, while pressing down, take slow and smooth diaphragmatic breaths in and out through the nose for a few moments, with your eyes closed if possible, and really focus on moving past your panic.

- Another acupressure point that is helpful for anxiety, and is particularly effective if you have a churning stomach or are feeling nauseous, is inside your forearm – three finger-widths up from the wrist crease, in between the two tendons. Follow a line down from your middle finger to your wrist crease, measure three finger-widths from here and you will hit the spot! As before, breathe rhythmically and slowly while pressing down on this point – either forearm will work.

If time permits, take 5–10 diaphragmatic breaths while pressing down on each acupressure point mentioned above, and focus your awareness on these areas – starting with the middle of the breastbone/sternum, then moving to the point just below your collarbones and finishing with the forearm points on both sides.

AFFIRMATION BREATHE

Affirmations are a form of positive self-talk and, when combined with slow, conscious breaths, can help by challenging and transforming negative thought patterns. Ideally you should practise affirmations up to three times a day for maximum benefit.

The affirmations given opposite are designed to encourage an extended outward breath. This is vital in quelling feelings of anxiety, as a longer exhalation will slow down the heart rate down and calm the body.

O Mindfully read the first part of the affirmation (in your head) while you breathe in.

O Then, as you read the words of the second part of the affirmation, breathe out.

O Repeat this 5–10 times, and really focus on how you express each affirmation. With each round, fill the affirmations with more conviction.

O As you build up your confidence with this technique, it's very effective to say the positive affirmations out loud while looking at yourself in a mirror. Try it – see how you feel. Does your posture change, as you start believing these words? Do you appear more confident?

O You can create your own affirmations, too. For instance, "I need more energy" or "I feel that I need more love, more rest". Be sure to write an affirmation that will inspire your day.

O You can also write these affirmations down on a small piece of card and pop it in your wallet or bag, to remind yourself to practise throughout the day.

Affirmation suggestions

Breathe in while reading the words on the left;
breathe out while reading the words on the right.

<u>INHALING</u>

<u>EXHALING</u>

I have resilience.   ○ ○ ○ ○ ○   I create space for these
negative feelings
and thoughts.

This feeling is   ○ ○ ○ ○ ○   I am far more than
temporary.   these feelings and
thoughts.

Breathing in,   ○ ○ ○ ○ ○   Breathing out, I begin
I find calm.   to feel lighter and my
mind is focused.

Deep breathing   ○ ○ ○ ○ ○   I release all of the
is my anchor.   stress, tension and
anxiety within me.

Breathing in,   ○ ○ ○ ○ ○   Breathing out, every
I smile.   single part of me softens
and finds stillness.

SHAPE-BREATHE

Many people find that it can be the waiting for an event or
appointment that causes them anxiety, but once they are
"in action" the anxiety melts away. So the following exercise
is great for those moments, such as waiting for a dental
appointment, when perhaps you start thinking about it in
more detail and your anxiety begins to rise. Practise this
technique for 5–10 minutes while you wait.

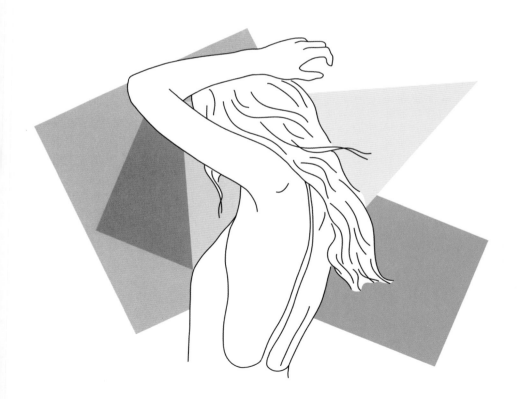

b e n e f i t s

Calms the nervous system

Refocuses the mind

Lowers stress

△ Look around you: what shapes can you see?

△ Are there any rectangles, squares or triangles in the room, for example? Any posters on the wall? You can do this exercise anywhere – from a bus stop to an office or a waiting room.

△ For a triangular shape, breathe in for a count of 3, hold the breath for a count of 3, then breathe out for a count of 3. Then repeat this 3 times.

Use the lines of each shape to guide the practice; do not force the breath, and make sure you are breathing in and out through the nose.

△ Then look around again and move on to the next shape you can see.

△ For a square or rectangle, use a count of 4: inhale for 4, hold the breath for 4, exhale for 4, hold for 4. Slow the breath down. Repeat 4 times before moving on.

"It ain't no use putting up your umbrella till it rains!"

ALICE CALDWELL RICE, AMERICAN AUTHOR

4

SLEEP

"No aspect of our biology is left unscathed by sleep deprivation."

DR. MATTHEW WALKER, ENGLISH NEUROSCIENTIST

We sleep for more than one-third of our lives: that's around 165,000,000 breaths, if we make it to the grand old age of 80. Sleep – and, more importantly, the quality of our sleep – is vital for a healthy, long life. Deep sleep helps restore our immune system, refines our metabolic state and improves our ability to learn and memorize.

The insightful book *Why We Sleep: The New Science of Sleep and Dreams* by Dr Matthew Walker, professor of neuroscience and psychology at the University of California, Berkeley, reveals:

> "Based on epidemiological studies of average sleep time, millions of individuals unwittingly spend years of their life in a sub-optimal state of psychological and physiological functioning, never maximizing their potential of mind or body due to their blind persistence in sleeping too little."

Which part of the brain is responsible for this life-saving deep sleep? It would seem that our sleep and respiratory centres share the same bed. The brainstem – especially the pons and medulla – is responsible for the rate at which we breathe involuntarily and also plays a special role in REM (Rapid Eye Movement) sleep; it sends signals to relax muscles that are essential for body posture and limb movements, so that we don't act out our dreams.

WHAT HAPPENS TO OUR BREATHING WHEN WE ARE ASLEEP?

Is there any link between the way we breathe and the quality of our sleep? Let's have a look at what happens to our breath while we are "out for the count".

Like other bodily functions, sleep happens in a cyclical fashion. There are four stages of sleep, and our breath pattern changes depending on which stage of sleep we are in. All four stages make up one cycle of sleep and can last anywhere up to 90 minutes. We should have roughly five or six cycles of non-REM and REM sleep during the night, with increasingly long, deep REM periods occurring toward morning. For a healthy body and mind, it is recommended that we sleep for an uninterrupted 8 hours every night.

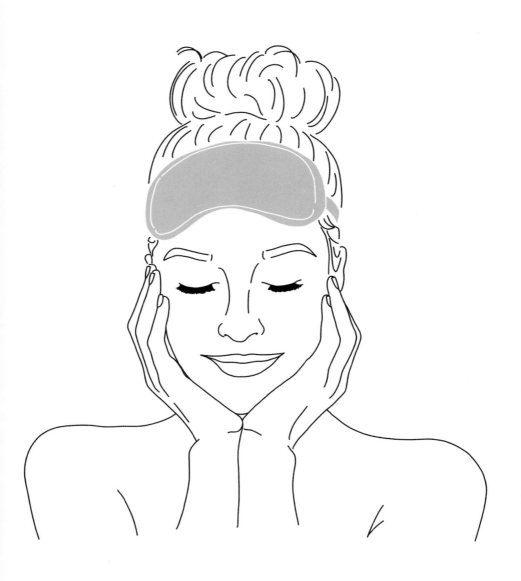

BREATHING STAGES

Here's how our breathing rate alters, along with other physiological changes, during each stage of slumber.

STAGE 1

During this relatively short transition from wakefulness to sleep, this non-REM sleep sees your breath rate slow down, your eye movements decelerate and your heartbeat find a more leisurely rhythm. Your muscles start to relax, with occasional twitches, and your brainwaves begin to slow.

STAGE 2

This non-REM sleep phase is the period of light sleep before you enter a deeper sleep. The breath finds an even slower rhythm, along with your heartbeat, and your muscles relax even further. Body temperature dips and your eye movements stop. Brainwave activity slows, but is marked by brief bursts of electrical activity; vast amounts of memory-processing are going on. You spend more of your repeated sleep cycles in stage-2 sleep than in other sleep phases.

STAGE 3

Non-REM sleep is the period of deep sleep that you need for your energies to feel restored in the morning. Your breath rate, along with your heartbeat, slows to its lowest level during this stage of sleeping. It occurs in longer periods during the first half of the night. Your muscles are relaxed and it may be a struggle to stir from this stage of slumber. Brainwaves become even slower.

STAGE 4

REM sleep is when your breath starts to quicken its rhythm and pace, becoming faster and irregular, which coincides with an increase in brainwave activity. In fact the brain is so active that it's close to a wakeful state. The blood pressure rises and the heart rate reaches a faster rhythm. It's a fascinating fact that during this stage your arms and legs become temporarily paralysed, and the muscles lose all their tone, which prevents you from acting out your dreams. Most of your dreaming occurs during REM sleep, although some can also occur in non-REM sleep. REM sleep is essential for creativity and intelligent decision-making.

"There is much that sleep can do that we in medicine currently cannot. So long as scientific evidence justifies it, we should make use of the powerful health tool that sleep represents in making our patients well."

DR MATTHEW WALKER, ENGLISH NEUROSCIENTIST

HOW BEST TO PREPARE OURSELVES FOR THE ULTIMATE KIP

It's important that we prepare ourselves for sleep. Much as we shower in the morning to wake ourselves up, so relaxing the body and mind before bed can help us on our way to a deeper, more restorative sleep.

With constant stimulation, artificial light, sound and screens, our modern lifestyles are making it increasingly difficult to enjoy a good night's sleep. Creating a sleep ritual that enables the mind to transition into the quiet, restorative nature of our evening allows us to enter a deep and nourishing sleep, which has a positive effect on our overall health and function.

If we encourage our body, breath and mind into a more rested state before we enter dreamland, it's more likely that we are going to reap the benefits that a night of quality sleep can bring. Relaxing the muscles, exercising the eyes and concentrating on slowing down our breath may be the perfect bridge to a first-class snooze.

The quality of my own sleep vastly improved after practising Yin Yoga. Vanessa Bridgeman is my all-time favourite Yin Yoga teacher. On the following pages, Vanessa shares her favourite super-calming Yin Yoga tips and poses to help you prepare for dreamland.

"Replenishing health with medicine is not as good as replenishing health with diet, but replenishing health with sleep is the best treatment of all."

CHINESE SAYING

WHY A YIN YOGA SEQUENCE CAN HELP YOU FIND THE ZZZZ

Yin Yoga is about finding postures without the activation or engagement of muscle tissue; instead the aim is to open fascia, tendons and ligaments of the body, staying for 1–5 minutes in each pose. On a more subtle level, we can use this practice to slow the fluctuation of thoughts, bringing our mind to the sensations in the body, which can soothe the mind and guide us away from all the busyness of our day. By slowing and elongating the breath, we can help promote the parasympathetic nervous system, readying ourselves fully for bed.

Yin Yoga is always best done at the end of the day – ideally, after a hot bath or shower, when the body is open and warm. On pages 84–86 are two poses you can enjoy to rid the body of accumulated tension, helping to promote undisturbed sleep.

THE YIN YOGA APPROACH

Find the structure of the shape/pose.

Wriggle around a bit. Allow yourself to explore it a little, as you settle in.

Find your edge. Always work with sensation, meeting the very edge of the physical body.

Build a fort, for support. Find the support you need, using props: pillows, blankets and so on. As the body recognizes the support, it will open and relax even further.

Stay a while: 1–5 minutes is best.

Surrender.

LEGS UP THE WALL

VIPARITA KARANI

If you have been on your feet all day, you can "reset"
the lower half of your body by resting your legs above
your head, using a wall as support. You can do this
exercise from your bed.

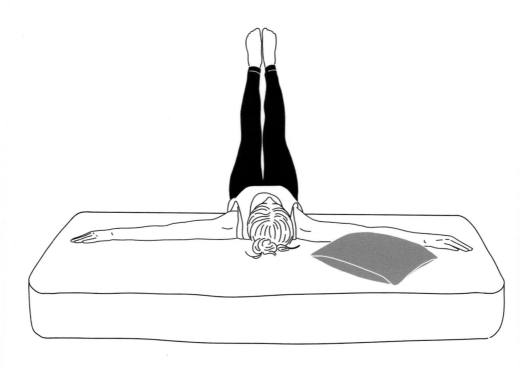

benefits

Takes the pressure off your heart to pump as hard,
and the heart rate slows

Improves circulation by drawing stagnant blood from
your legs to the lower torso

Reduces swelling and fatigue in your legs

O Begin by placing your hips
as close to the wall (or the bed's
headboard) as possible and then
lying back, swinging your legs
up as you lie on your back. You
may like some support, such as a
blanket or pillow, under your head
and/or lower back.

O Relax all the muscles through your
legs and body, perhaps bringing
your arms out wide. Or place your
arms over your head, with a
bend in the elbows to relax
your shoulders.

O Stay in this pose for 5–15 minutes.
You might enjoy taking your legs
wide or bringing the soles of the
feet together and the knees open.
Respond to your body as you
listen closely to its needs.

SEATED DANGLE

Dangling brings about the qualities that we look to cultivate throughout any shape in Yin Yoga practice: introspection, yielding and letting go.

---

b e n e f i t s

Alleviates stress and anxiety

Therapeutic for high blood pressure

O Sitting on the edge of the bed, find this pose by first placing your feet hip-width apart. Begin to roll your body forward over your legs, allowing the torso to rest on your legs and letting your arms, shoulders and head hang heavy.

O Ensure that your feet stay relaxed and, as you let your awareness turn inward, feel your belly rise into your thighs on the next inhalation. Relax other parts of your body that may tighten as you exhale, softening your jaw and brow.

O Dangle here for 3 minutes or so and let the day melt away – allow your breath to soften and slow down.

NB: Avoid dangling if you have back issues.

MIDNIGHT-HOUR BREATHS

When we fall asleep, we can only hope to wake in the morning feeling fully revitalized and energized, after an undisturbed eight hours' rest. Unfortunately, more often than not we will wake at some point during the night.

A 2017 study by Canadian health experts calculated that people spend seven years of their lives lying awake at night, trying to fall asleep – that's around 43 million breaths. What if we used these breaths to coax us back into a dreamland? Here are some tried-and-tested breath techniques to help lull you back to sleep, if you wake during the night.

"We spend nearly 51,100,000 breaths in our lifetimes trying to get to sleep."

SUPER SLUMBER-HERO

Sleeping well is a superpower and, for a large proportion of my life, I felt like I was a "40-winks wonder-woman". It was my only gift, which was sadly snatched from me after the birth of my first (and second) child. I suddenly suffered bouts of insomnia, and restless nights became the norm. I felt that I had entered a dark land, where my nights were overactive and I wandered through my days in a semi-narcoleptic state.

On a positive note, and retrospectively, those nights also served as the perfect playground for me to experiment with breathing exercises to help my brain into a sleepier state. After a good six months of trying everything, from coordinating my inhales and exhales with my partner's snoring pattern, to practising every breathwork exercise under the moon, here are my favourite breathing techniques to help induce sleep.

———

"A ruffled mind makes a restless pillow."
CHARLOTTE BRONTË, ENGLISH NOVELIST AND POET

BEDTIME BREATHE

Dr Ben Marshall, respiratory consultant at Southampton University, Hampshire, UK, highly recommends the following breathing technique to help you back into sleep mode.

---

benefits

Calms the mind

Resets the nervous system

Stimulates the parasympathetic nervous system

The breath-hold releases nitric oxide

Easy to remember

O Lie in a comfortable position.

O To prepare, engage in a few rounds of muscle tensing and releasing. Inhale as you tense all the muscles of the body. Squeeze your hands into fists, squeeze the muscles of your legs and arms in toward the bones. Tense all the muscles in your face.

O Exhaling through the mouth, relax all your muscles.

O Repeat a few times.

O Keep space between the top and bottom teeth, and place the tip of your tongue to the hard palate of your mouth.

O Breathe 3–4–5, as follows: Breathe in through the nose for a count of 3. Hold the breath in for a count of 4. Breathe out through the mouth for a count of 5. Repeat for at least 10 rounds or until you drift off.

YAWNING BREATHE

This is really simple and will trick the body into thinking it's more than ready for some deep sleep.

If you wake up in the night, simply start yawning. You may have to pretend at first, but soon a real yawn will emerge. Do this until you have given ten proper yawns. Get your entire body involved, too: stretch the arms and legs while the mouth is wide, then relax the limbs as the mouth closes. You will soon start to appreciate all the physiological benefits that a yawn can bring, including cooling the brain and relaxing the body.

EYES WIDE SHUT

Ever noticed how babies blink their eyes as they fight to fall asleep? What if this slow blinking routine is an innate intelligence, guiding them into a deeper sleep? This is a breath and eye coordination exercise to practise, one which will hopefully lull you back to sleep.

benefits

Promotes feelings of calm

Reduces heart rate and lowers blood pressure

○ Breathing in through the nose slowly, blink your eyes open.

○ Breathing out through the nose slowly, blink your eyes closed.

○ Repeat and, even if you feel you are drifting off, keep blinking your eyes open as you breathe in and shut as you breathe out, for a few more rounds. Eventually you should reach the point where it's a real effort to open your eyes.

○ You can bring a breath count into this if you want to focus the mind.

○ Breathing in, blink your eyes open for 1...2...3...4.

○ Breathing out, blink your eyes shut for 1...2...3...4.

B IS...FOR BREATHE

This is quite an unusual technique, which came to me in the early hours, and has worked for me during many a sleepless night. The consistent slow breathing in and out of the left nostril will help activate the parasympathetic nervous system and cool the body down – a great precursor for sleep. Add the B-word game to this exercise to keep the mind from overthinking.

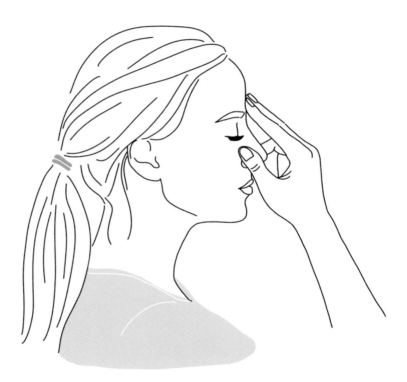

benefits

Focuses the mind

Prevents overthinking about daily worries

Helps you drift off to sleep

O With your eyes softly closed and your jaw relaxed, find a comfortable position lying down, either on your back or on your side.

O Practise some Left-Nostril Breathing: block off your right nostril by 90 per cent (using one finger pressed to the outside of the right nostril, with a tiny space for an airway) and breathe in and out slowly through your left nostril only. You may find that your left nostril is slightly blocked – this means the right nostril is your dominant breathing nostril (so you don't completely block it).

O Breathing in through your left nostril slowly and smoothly, think of a word

beginning with B (for instance, "breathe").

O Breathing out though the left nostril, try and visualize this word (someone breathing out).

O Breathing in slowly through the left nostril, think of another word beginning with B (for instance, "banana").

O Breathing out through the left nostril, visualize this word.

O Find a different word with the same letter and visualize it, for each inhalation and exhalation.

HEARTBEAT BREATHE

Using the internal metronome of the heartbeat can be an
effective way to lull you into a peaceful slumber.

---

benefits

Quietens the mind

Slows the breath rate down

Lowers blood pressure

Allows the body to enter a rest-and-digest state

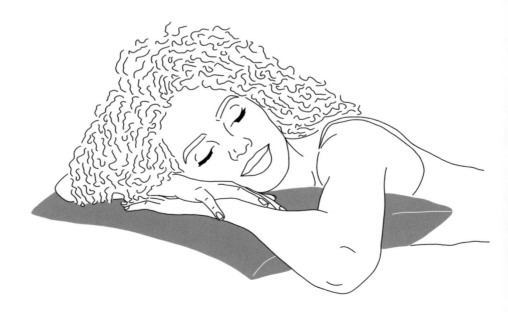

○ Lie on your belly or on the side of the body that feels most comfortable.

○ Feel a sense of "letting go" and allow the body to "sink" into the mattress.

○ If you are lying on your left side, slip your left hand under your pillow, so it is parallel with your left ear; this will apply a little pressure between your pillow and your ear. (And vice versa if you are lying on your right side.)

○ Bring your awareness to your left (or right) ear, or the space in between the pillow and your hand. You should be able to hear the beat of your heart. Use your heartbeat as a guide (it will be beating at 60–75 beats per minute); this will help you set the pace of your breath.

○ Breathe 6–2–8, as follows:

○ Breathe in through the nose for 6 heartbeats.

○ Hold the breath for 2 heartbeats.

○ Breathe out through the nose for 8 heartbeats.

○ You may notice that your heartbeat slows down after a few rounds. And... hopefully you will drift off mid-count.

If your mind is still fighting for your attention, you can bring your awareness to the silence between each beat of the heart. Focus on this for a few more breaths. The extension of the exhalation will activate the parasympathetic nervous system and the focus on the heartbeat will take your mind off your thoughts. For some, the soft beating of the heart can have a soothing effect.

SPIRAL-BREATHE FOR SLEEP

Starting at the centre, follow the spiral line with your eye gaze, inhaling and exhaling when prompted.

There should be no breath-holding. Repeat this 5–10 times, then close your eyes, still visualizing the spiral. Repeat for 5 more cycles. This should help you drift off to sleep very quickly.

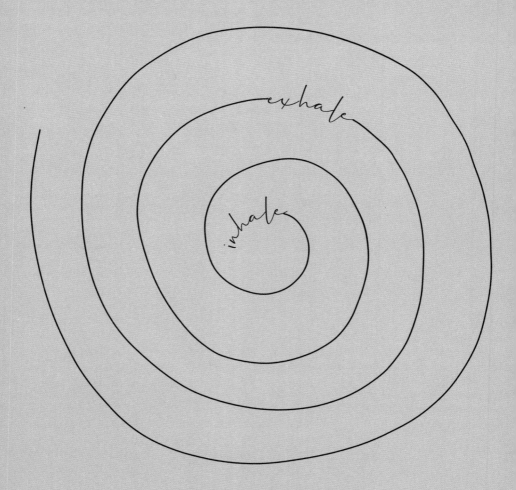

DREAM-BREATHE

Stan Cortes, another favourite yoga teacher of mine,
kindly shared this technique with me while I was writing
this book. It's very simple and extremely effective.
It helped to calm down my overactive mind and sent
me off to sleep in just a few rounds.

benefits

Helps calm the nervous system

Relaxes the mind

Promotes a deep, undisturbed sleep

○ Lie down in your most comfortable position and gently inhale through the nose.

○ Exhale fully through the mouth, then switch.

○ Inhale through the mouth and exhale through the nose.

○ Practise this very calmly and silently. Be present. Repeat for 5–10 rounds.

○ You can also apply acupressure for 1–2 rounds. There's a great acu-point either side of your ankle bone, which helps activate the diaphragm and stimulate the vagus nerve, which is known for helping your nervous system relax. With your index finger and thumb, press the underside of either side of the base of your ankle bone – it will feel tender when you're at the right spot – while you repeat the next round. Then drift off...

5

SOJOURNS

"The real voyage of discovery consists not in seeking new landscapes, but in having new eyes."

MARCEL PROUST, FRENCH NOVELIST

Surprisingly, the average person will spend just under three years (around 18 million breaths) of their life away from home in other destinations – be that on a holiday, an adventure or a weekend sojourn.

While the thought of escaping from the daily grind can bring feelings of excitement, with the hope of a break and relaxation on the horizon, sometimes adapting to a new climate and culture can also be stressful.

Even if you are not travelling far, simply making your way to your destination can have a plethora of challenges: the endless waiting at train stations and airports, navigating your way around a new city, driving on the "wrong side" of the road or trekking across new landscapes can all create minor (and sometimes major) havoc for your nervous system. And if you are travelling long-haul, waking in a different time zone can cause chaos to your circadian rhythm (your body's internal clock), which can leave you feeling depleted of vital energy.

When you book your next break, be sure to pack a few breath techniques as well, to help rebalance your energies.

CHECK-IN BREATHE

This is a great technique to use in the departure lounge or waiting room, before boarding a plane or train. A few conscious breaths will help induce feelings of calm and stillness.

It is best practised sitting down, with the support of the back of a chair, if possible. However, it can also help pass some time if you find yourself standing in a long queue.

"A change is as good as a rest."

ENGLISH PROVERB

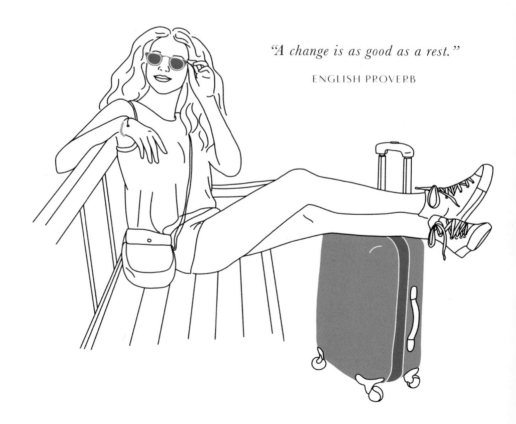

b e n e f i t s

Activates the parasympathetic nervous system

Calms the mind

Brings your awareness back to the present moment

Staves off boredom

○ Relax your face; using your index and middle fingers, gently massage your face for a minute, focusing on the jaw, which is often a hotspot for tension. Allow space between your top and bottom jaws and place the tip of your tongue to the roof of your mouth. Take a few nasal breaths.

○ Place your hands behind your back, so that the palms of your hands rest on your back, just above your hip bones. The tips of your middle fingers should touch, for the hands to be in a good position.

○ Take a few breaths and notice which side of your body is moving more. Is the left or the right side moving more on the inhalation?

○ Maybe your body is moving in an even rhythm. Just be curious about how each breath moves the body.

○ Slowing your breath down now to an easy rhythm, inhale through the nose and become aware of the back of your body expanding into the palms of your hands on the inhale. Breathe 5–3–5, as follows:

○ Breathe in through the nose for a count of 5.

○ Hold for a count of 3.

○ Breathe out through the nose for a count of 5.

○ Repeat as the diaphragm descends, expanding the belly and lower back.

ON-BOARD BREATHE

Once on board, this is an effective "body scan" technique that will enable you to let go of unwanted tension and will prepare you for a comfortable trip. Removing your shoes lets your feet and body feel more grounded – even if you are about to "take off".

---

benefits

Calms the nervous system

Cultivates present moment awareness

Quietens an overactive mind

Re-establishes a diaphragmatic breath

○ Inhale through the nose and hold this book at your belly button. Exhale fully through the mouth.

○ Uncross your legs and ankles. Feel your thighs relax into your chair, letting your legs feel heavy. Feel your shins and calves become heavier and visualize the soles of your feet.

○ Imagine your soles sinking into the surface beneath them; bring your awareness to the ball of your big toe and apply a little weight to this area.

○ Feel a slight pressure between the ball of your toe and the floor. Now, spread all your toes wide, lifting them and then placing them back to the floor.

BREATHE AND READ

Breathe in through the nose for as long it takes you to read this sentence.

Breathe out slowly and softly through the mouth until your eyes reach the very end of this line.

Take another breath in through the nose, reading all the way along this line.

Breathe out slowly and softly through the mouth until your eyes reach the very end of this sentence. Repeat.

"It is better to travel well than to arrive."

BUDDHA

BREATH OF FIRE

Travelling, and being in a different location, can sometimes divert our normal eating habits and disrupt our digestive system. This breath practice can help you to stimulate the digestive system and boost your energy, too.

Breath of Fire has a quick, rhythmic and continuous pace and should only be performed once you have established a healthy "diaphragmatic breath" (see pages 16–20). It is best practised in the morning on an empty stomach. It's important to note that Breath of Fire is <u>not</u> hyperventilation.

---

benefits

Strengthens the digestive system

Balances the nervous system

Purifies the respiratory system

Releases natural energy within the body

NB: Refrain from practising this exercise if you are pregnant, menstruating, have high blood pressure, stomach ulcers or have suffered from a stroke/heart disease.

O Sit with a tall spine and your chin parallel to the floor. Your jaw should be relaxed.

O Focus on your navel.

O Expel (with a little force) all the air through your nose, and feel your navel draw back toward the spine.

O Inhale through the nose with pace.

O Exhale in one short blast through the nostrils.

O The inhale should come in on its own, almost silently. Now start to pick up the pace. Inhale and then…

O Exhale again in one short blast through the nostrils – the upper abdominal muscles pull in and up on the exhalation.

O Repeat. The breath should sound like a steam train gaining pace. The pace should be quick and you will feel energy build in the system. You may notice some tingling sensations and light-headedness, which is normal. Close your eyes and take your internal gaze to the point in between your eyebrows.

O Repeat for 1–3 minutes and notice how you feel.

"No one realizes how beautiful it is to travel until he comes home and rests his head on his old, familiar pillow."

LIN YUTANG, CHINESE WRITER

BIOPHILIA BREATHE

The "biophilia hypothesis" suggests that humans have an innate tendency to seek connections with nature and other forms of life. If you have arrived in a new city or landscape, be sure to visit a natural spot as soon as time permits. Spending time in nature has proven health benefits, including helping to reduce our levels of cortisol – the "stress hormone". Practising breathing exercises within a natural environment can help you recharge your system. Nature is our greatest teacher, after all.

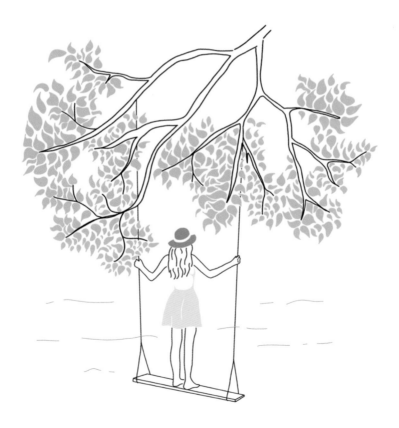

BREATHING ROOMS

The Hintze Hall at London's Natural History Museum is one of my favourite "breathing rooms". In collaboration with the London yoga studio East of Eden, I was asked to create a nature-themed breath routine to teach to 170 people, in the space of the largest lungs in the world – those of the blue whale skeleton, which is suspended from the ceiling of this magnificent Victorian gallery.

This incredible teaching experience in the nave of this "cathedral to nature" – which houses 80 million specimens and is widely acknowledged as the world's most important natural-history collection – further fuelled my passion for breathwork and my appreciation of the natural world.

As I embarked on a personal research mission and discovered innumerable breathing patterns within the animal kingdom, I began to wonder how many ancient breath practices had evolved from observing the way other mammals breathe. There are many yogic practices that refer to animals – for instance, Lion's Breath, Crocodile Pose, Frog Pose, Fish Pose, Cat and Cow, to name just a few.

———

"Intelligence is based on how efficient a species became at doing the things they need to survive."

CHARLES DARWIN, ENGLISH NATURALIST

THE AIR WE BREATHE

All land dwellers share the same air, but we all breathe in unique and fascinating ways. Remarkably, a few ocean inhabitants can survive at a depth of up to 8,000m (26,240ft), and other marine creatures are inspirational breath-holders, too. But who took the very first breath here on Earth?

According to zoologists, the pioneer of respiration was the mighty sea sponge. It could have performed the very first "breath" as it helped to release a flood of oxygen into the (once oxygen-less) ocean, around 700 million years ago. We may have the sea sponge to thank for our respiration origins – some species even look like lungs!

A short while after the sea sponge, came prehistoric earthworms and insects, which evolved to breathe entirely through their skin and exoskeletons. From the lung-less sea spiders that can only breathe through their legs, to the upside-down hanging sloths, which have special muscles that attach their lower organs to their ribs in order to take a breath, the breathing patterns within the natural world (about which we will learn more shortly) are boundless. And where does this breath or, more importantly, this life-giving gas – oxygen – come from?

The majority of the world's oxygen supply comes from tiny ocean plants called phytoplankton (or diatoms) that live near the water's surface. Trees are the second-largest supplier of the vital oxygen that we breathe (and the chief absorber of carbon dioxide), with up to 20 per cent produced by the Amazon rainforest. This is why it's paramount that we protect, love and care for our oceans and forests. The oxygen within the air you have just inhaled while reading this sentence has been produced by either one of these magical, life-giving habitats.

Forests and oceans are our "life force", so much so that recent studies have shown that even spending a short amount of time in a natural habitat can have an extremely positive effect on our overall health and wellbeing. (It's been reported that some doctors in Scotland are now issuing "nature prescriptions" to help treat mental illness, diabetes, heart disease, stress and other conditions.)

Simply looking at pictures of green spaces can help calm our nervous system, too. In a 2012 study conducted in waiting rooms at a Dutch hospital, patients who were exposed to either real plants or pictures of plants experienced less stress, compared to people who saw neither.

Inspired by the natural world, the following exercises are best experienced outdoors, in an abundance of fresh air. However, should you be indoors, you can still reap all the benefits that these breathing practices can bring.

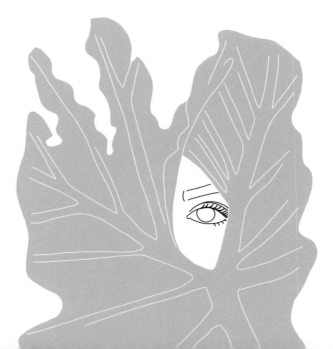

BEES

"If you compare an athlete, the bee and the hummingbird, the bee is the champion of oxygen delivery."

SCOTT KIRKTON, PROFESSOR OF BIOLOGICAL
SCIENCES, UNION COLLEGE

Bees are not only the most important species for human survival (they pollinate 70 of the 100 or so crop species that feed 90 per cent of the world), they are a breathing phenomenon. Bees have neither a pair of lungs nor a nose. Instead, bees draw in oxygen through holes in their bodies known as "spiracles" and pump the oxygen through a system of increasingly tiny tubes (tracheae) that deliver oxygen directly to their tissues and muscles.

The speedy wingbeats of bees stir up vibrations in the air, causing us to hear the buzz. And we can mimic that buzz, or hum, of the bee and reap some sweet rewards.

HUM YOUR WAY TO HAPPINESS

You can practise the traditional Bhramari or Bee Breath (see pages 60–61), but simple humming can also have positive effects on the body and mind. Humming can improve air flow between the sinuses and the nasal cavity, helping to protect the health of your sinuses.

---

benefits

Calms a busy mind

Relaxes the nervous system

Slows down the breath rate

Lowers blood pressure

Enhances focus

Extended exhalation stimulates the vagus nerve

O Allow space between your top and bottom teeth and relax your face. Inhale deeply through the nose while thinking of a (favourite) tune, and, when you are ready to exhale, hum your tune until your breath runs out.

O Make sure you use the entire range of your breath; so inhale slowly and fully and hum away, using the full length of your exhalation.

THE PUFFER FISH

Within moments of sensing a nearby threat, the puffer fish can swell up into a spiny sphere. While it may seem as if these creatures are holding their breath as they inflate, they can actually breathe completely efficiently in their puffed-up state.

It comes as no surprise that this breath exercise is the perfect antidote for when our nervous system feels under attack. Inspired by the puffer fish, and by a much-loved book called *Perfect Breathing* by Al Lee and Don Campbell, this technique will allow you to dive into a state of calm. Make sure you have established deep diaphragmatic breathing (see page 20) before attempting this exercise.

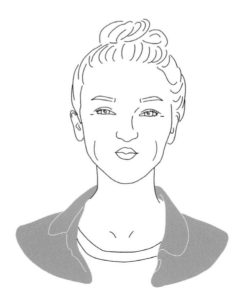

benefits

Effective for anyone suffering from anxiety
or mild panic attacks

By pursing your lips and inflating your cheeks, you'
put pressure on the vagus nerve in the back of your
throat, which can curtail any telltale symptoms of
anxiety, such as sweating, a racing heart and nausea

Helps you to feel calm and present

Quietens the mind

○ Connect with your inner puffer fish. Breathe...beginning with a full exhalation.

○ Then fill your lungs with a slow inhalation from the belly to the top of the lungs.

○ Inflate your cheeks and purse your lips, as if blowing out through a straw, as you exhale through the mouth. Keep your cheeks inflated as you exhale for a count of 10 (repeating in your mind, "1 – one thousand, 2 – two thousand" until you reach 10).

○ Close your mouth and begin again with a slow, deep inhale through the nose.

○ Then exhale through the mouth, with your cheeks inflated for the full duration of the exhale.

○ Repeat for 3–5 minutes or until you are feeling calm.

THE "GORILLA CHILLER"

The upper part of the respiratory system, after the brain, consists of the nasal cavity, trachea (windpipe) and larynx (front of the throat). Just above is an interesting bone called the hyoid, which is the only "floating" bone in the body. The position of the larynx and hyoid bone is unique to humans and works in perfect unison with the tongue – making humans the main "chit-chatterers" of the animal world. Without this unique positioning, we would still be hooting, grunting and "ahhhingg" like our gorilla cousins. No other animal has a larynx low enough to produce sounds as complex as those of our ancient ancestors. Perhaps the day the larynx dropped, and Neanderthals started to use oxygen for "chatting", was the day we started to lose a vital connection to our respiratory system. Possibly it was then that we began to "waste our breath".

Channelling our ancestral "inner gorilla" can help us flex our vocal cords, reconnecting us with a primal sound. This breath exercise can often bring on a bout of the giggles, too, which can also be a welcome workout for the diaphragm.

b e n e f i t s

Peps up energy levels

Clears stagnant energy around the throat and vocal cords

Aids the "rest-and-digest" response

Challenges your comfort zone

○ Find a peaceful spot out in nature. This exercise is best done alone!

○ Stand or sit in a comfortable position.

○ Inhale slowly and deeply through the nostrils, taking a deep belly breath in; then take in a little more air, to fill the upper chest with air.

○ On the exhalation, open your mouth nice and wide and make a gorilla-like sound: "Ahhhhhh". Continue with this sound until the breath and the sound comes to a natural end.

○ Now you can bring your "gorilla hands" into play. Gorillas use their palms, not their fists, to beat their chests. Bringing both hands to your upper chest, place your palms flat there, just below the collarbone. Close

your eyes, if that makes it easier to feel physical sensations in the body.

○ Inhale slowly through the nose.

○ Open your mouth, breathing out, and make a low gorilla-like "Ahhhhhh" sound as you exhale. Beat the palms of your hands on the upper chest, just below your collarbone.

○ Take a few resting breaths – in and out through the nose – between each round, and notice any physical sensations. Some people feel energy moving in their upper chest and vibrations below the collarbone, and sometimes mild vibrations in the throat.

○ Finish the practice by closing your eyes and placing the hands over the heart centre. See if any feelings arise.

TORTOISE-BREATHE

The slowest breather on Earth, the Galápagos tortoise, is also one of the longest-living animals. Its breath rate is four breaths a minute (compared with an average of 12 breaths per minute for humans). We could hypothesize that by slowing down our breath rate, we could also slow down our lives.

The tortoise, which is a symbol of longevity in China, was the inspiration for a Qigong (pronounced "chi-kung") meditative breath practice, known as Tortoise Breathing or "kuei hsi" – "swallowing the breath" – which aims to mimic the slow, deliberate breathing of this land-dwelling reptile. This is a much-favoured technique in the medical world. A senior respiratory consultant in New Delhi, Dr Partha Pratim Bose, recommends regular practice of it, to help slow the heart rate and calm the mind.

This is a great exercise to help you reconnect with your breath and your surroundings. Choose a warm sunny spot – maybe on a beach, in a field or deep in forest. Using the Tortoise Breathing technique, with time and practice you should be able to slow down your breathing rate to around 4–5 breaths per minute.

Increases energy levels

Calms the mind

Lowers blood pressure

Reduces inflammation and balances pH levels

O Start either sitting or lying down on your back. Let your body relax into the ground. Take a long breath, inhaling slowly and deeply through your mouth until you feel the air inside your throat.

O "Swallow" your breath by taking the air down your throat. Imagine that you are swallowing a small piece of your favourite food. (Note that the swallowing acts as a breath-hold, as you cannot breathe and swallow simultaneously.)

O Exhale deeply and slowly through the nostrils, not your mouth, immediately after swallowing.

O Repeat this inhale–swallow–exhale cycle 7 times.

O Following the seventh breath, move your tongue around the inside of your mouth to collect the saliva and swallow several times. If you find the swallowing part of this exercise uncomfortable (it can take a little practice), you can bring your breath rate down to a more tortoise-like, less hare-like pace of 5 breaths per minute simply by breathing in for a count of 6, then breathing out for a count of 6.

O If you are practising this at home, you may like to bring yourself into Child's Pose and imagine that you are a tortoise! Simply come to a kneeling position and bow your head to the floor, with your arms resting beside your thighs, palms facing upward.

THE BODHI-TREE BREATHE

("40 breaths to calm you")

With the fast pace of modern life you perhaps won't have the time, or the inclination, to sit and meditate under a tree for 40 days. Siddhartha Gautama, the Buddha, achieved an enlightened state after completing this 40-day meditation marathon – although life was possibly a lot less distracting in 450 BCE.

Finding time for 40 breaths (about 5 minutes) is a lot more feasible and will still enable you to reconnect with your breath, a meditative state and the natural environment.

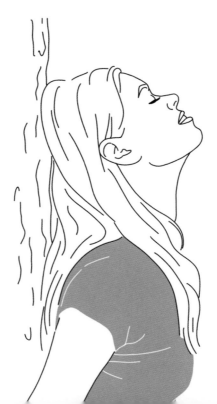

benefits

Calms the nervous system

Quietens the mind

Helps you connect with nature

Promotes a meditative state of mind

○ Find a tree, preferably in a forest, park or peaceful garden. Choose a tree that you feel looks strong, wise and inviting. Have your back supported by the tree trunk, whether you are sitting or standing.

○ Place your hands on your lower belly and feel the trunk of the tree providing support for your back. Close your eyes and feel your connection to this unique tree. Take a moment to reflect upon how unique it is: the only tree on the entire planet to have grown in this individually beautiful way. Then bring your awareness to all the qualities about yourself that make you completely unique. Be in awe that there is no one exactly like you.

○ Breathe slowly and fully for 40 breaths, counting the breaths inwardly, if this is helpful. Allow the inhalations to be the odd numbers and the exhalations to be the even numbers. For instance: "Inhale 1, exhale 2, inhale 3, exhale 4", and so on. Work your way up to 40 (this will be 20 full breaths).

○ Repeat again.

○ When you have finished, take a few more breaths, feeling the earth beneath you, the tree supporting you, and listen to the sounds around you.

○ Slowly blink open your eyes. Do your surroundings look brighter or clearer? Do you feel calmer, more connected?

6

LEARNING

*"Man is most nearly himself when he achieves
the seriousness of a child at play."*

HERACLITUS, GREEK PHILOSOPHER

During our lifetime most of us will spend around 13 years (that's about 80 million breaths) at school, college or university. The first years of school can be both exciting and nerve-racking for children. From running free as a toddler, surrounded by close family or carers, to suddenly being in a small classroom with lots of new faces and being told to "sit down", "be still", "keep quiet" and focus on reading, writing or counting can go against our creative nature of wishing to move and play.

With the pressure on many educational institutions to perform to an outstanding level (with limited resources), it is no wonder the school environment can be a melting pot for stress and anxiety. Seeing my own son's transition from home to school, and witnessing first-hand all the pressures this can bring (to both pupils and teachers), I was inspired to develop a School Breathe programme. This is a selection of easy-to-learn breathing techniques that encourages pupils and teachers to spend a few minutes at the beginning of the day focusing on their breathing and starting their learning in a peaceful frame of mind.

The following exercises have been designed for children, but adults and teachers love them, too; you don't have to own a pair of young lungs in order to enjoy them – in fact it can be therapeutic to invite a sense of play and imagination back into our lives, whatever our age.

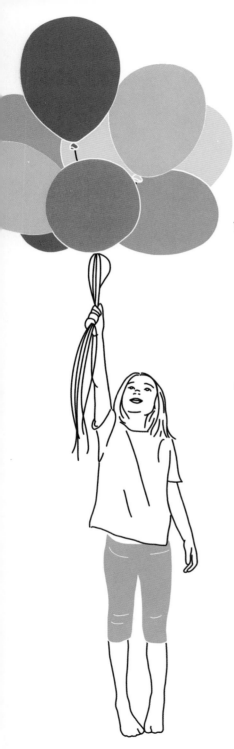

BALLOON
BREATHE

This is a very popular breathing technique, for children and adults. If you are a parent, carer, family member or teacher, you can read the following instructions out loud to your children and, over time, they will be able to practise on their own.

With a large proportion of the school day spent seated, I encourage children to stand while practising this breath exercise. However, it is also an effective technique to practise lying down in bed, just before sleep.

―――――――――

"The breathing techniques are so relaxing and help me empty my mind and feel refreshed."

KEAN, AGED NINE

b e n e f i t s

Builds breath awareness

Brings children into the present moment

Cultivates healthy breathing habits

Encourages a belly breath

Calms the nervous system

○ If standing, place your feet firmly on the ground. If lying down, make sure that your head is supported with a cushion or pillow.

○ Place the palms of your hands just below your belly button (or "breathing button").

○ Take a slow breath in through the nose and see if you notice your belly rising with the hands – imagine a colourful balloon filling with air.

○ Breathe out slowly through the nose: your belly should deflate, just like a balloon losing air, and return to its resting position.

○ Breathing in, imagine the balloon in your belly rising up a little higher now. Can you feel, or see, your belly rise?

○ Breathing out, feel your belly lower to its starting position.

○ Now let's count (increase or decrease the count, depending on the child's ability – younger children may only be able to breathe in for a count of 3).

○ Breathing in 1...2...3...4.

○ Breathing out 1...2...3...4.

○ Repeat for 5 rounds.

HOT-CHOCOLATE BREATHE

Children's imaginations are vast and they love to use imagery to learn, play and breathe. This is a popular exercise for all ages. If there are some children who aren't keen on hot chocolate, ask them to imagine their favourite warm drink instead.

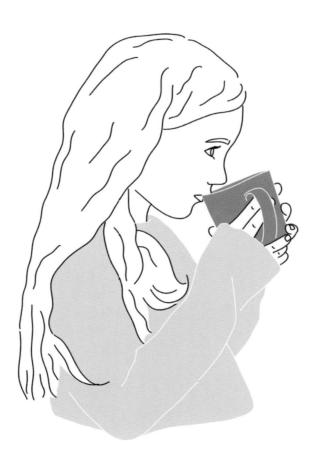

benefits

Exercises the imagination

Extending the exhalation triggers a relaxation response

Brings children into the present moment

Cultivates a fun relationship with breathwork

Quietens the mind

Calms the nervous system

○ Imagine you are holding a mug of the most delicious hot chocolate. The warmth of the mug brings heat to your hands.

○ Bring the imaginary cup up to just under your nose. Take a long inhale through the nose, and imagine smelling all the delicious, rich flavours of chocolate.

○ Gently breathe out through your lips, as you cool the hot chocolate down. Imagine you can see steam drifting away from the mug as you breathe out.

○ Breathe in slowly, as you allow the scent of the hot chocolate to enter your nostrils.

○ Slowly breathe out through your lips, as you cool the hot chocolate down a little more.

○ Repeat one more time, breathing in slowly through the nose and breathing out fully through the mouth. Your hot chocolate is (nearly) ready to drink...

○ You can end the breath exercise here or, if the children are slightly older and have a longer attention span, you can add a Marshmallow Breath-Hold (see overleaf).

MARSHMALLOW
BREATH-HOLD

Just before you take a sip...

You look at the huge marshmallow floating on top of
the hot chocolate, and you take it slowly and carefully
with your fingertips – it feels light and fluffy. This
marshmallow is HUGE. You open your mouth wide
and pop the marshmallow into your mouth. Hold the
breath: 1...2...3... Imagine big marshmallow cheeks.
Breathe out through the nose, breathe in through the
nose, breathe out through the nose. Now chew your
marshmallow well and swallow it.

Now you can take a big sip of your hot chocolate.

FROG-SQUAT BREATHE

During my time teaching I've noticed how many children
find it difficult to hold the squat position for even a few
breaths. Stiff hips, weakened quadriceps and low tone
in the abdominal muscles are all too common in today's
classrooms, where being told to sit down and keep still for
five hours a day has become the norm.

Squatting is one of the most effective ways to tone the entire
lower body. It works the quadriceps, hamstrings, glutes and
calf muscles, and it strengthens the lower back and core
muscles. It's also the perfect opportunity to establish a healthy
breath. If the hands adopt the prayer position, this allows for
a lengthening of the thoracic spine and makes room for the
diaphragm to move freely, so this is an ideal position in which
to connect with a full breath.

In Western cultures, we rarely see someone in a full squat pose
outside the yoga studio (unless they are a toddler). In the East
and Africa people of all ages still adopt the squat position for
chatting, eating, working and socializing.

We have the ancient Egyptians to thank for all the chairs
that we sit on today, for they invented the throne-like "chair
with a backrest". This served the Egyptians well, when sitting

for elaborate feasts and the occasional important meeting. However, we can hypothesize that it was when we started to embrace sitting down on chairs for schooling, work and downtime that we began to lose our healthy posture.

The seated chair position promotes poor posture, and therefore poor breathing. To adopt these unhealthy habits from such a young age can have a ripple effect on our wellbeing later in life. It's essential that we remind our children (and ourselves) to practise the "natural seat" position more often, to enable us to strengthen our muscles and our respiratory system.

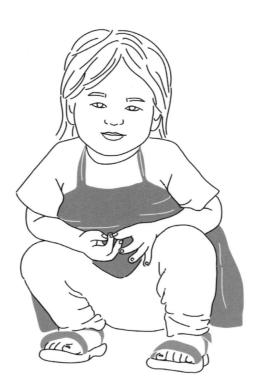

benefits

Stretches the ankles and lower back

Improves the respiratory system

Tones the core muscles

Stimulates the digestive system

Promotes a healthy breath and improves posture

○ Start in a standing position, feet hip-width apart, pointing outward about 45 degrees.

○ Gently roll your torso down over your thighs and let your head, arms and hands hang low toward the floor.

○ Bend your legs so that your hands can touch the ground.

○ Using your hands to stabilize you, lower your buttocks toward the floor until you enter a squat position, keeping your heels and the balls of your feet planted on the floor. (Lift your heels, if this is easier for you.)

○ Have your hands together in prayer position, elbows inside your knees.

○ Make sure this is comfortable for your feet, knees and thighs. Give this pose patience and practice.

○ Now take a deep, slow breath in through the nose: 1...2...3...4...

○ And gently breathe out through the mouth: 1...2...3...4...

○ Repeat for 5–10 breaths. Notice if you feel it easier to breathe into the belly in this position.

NB: Avoid this pose if you have issues with your Achilles tendon, ankles or knees.

OCTOPUS BREATHE

My research into how animals breathe reintroduced me to the mesmeric octopus. This fascinating animal breathes both in and out of its siphon-like mouth. This pumps water in and around the gills where it extracts oxygen from the water, which it then pumps through all three of its hearts and around its entire body.

This is a popular exercise for 7–9-year-olds and a great way to get kids to connect with their breath using their "tentacle" arms. It can also bring children's awareness to the oceanic depths of their breath: taking breaths while focusing on four different areas of the body shows them how their entire torso moves with each breath.

benefits

Enhances breath awareness

Promotes a full breath

Focuses the mind

Builds body awareness

Encourages learning to breathe through play

○ Either practise this standing or find a comfortable seat. Have your feet firmly planted on the floor and the spine tall, so there is space between your lower ribs and hips.

○ Place the palms of your hands (or tips of your tentacles!) below your belly button.

○ Take a slow breath in, through the nose. Imagine and feel your belly rising as you take the air deep into your lungs. If your imagination is running wild today, you can even visualize that your belly is the head, or "mantle", of an octopus: bulbous, full and rising as you breathe in.

○ Make an O-shape with your mouth and breathe out slowly through it, listening to the sound of the breath as it leaves your body, just like the ocean.

○ Inhale and exhale again like this, without moving your hands.

○ Now take each hand to either side of your body, between the top of your hips and the bottom of your ribcage.

○ Take a deep breath in through the nose and notice how your body expands outward into your hands as you breathe in. Then make your mouth into an O-shape again, and breathe out through it. Slow it down. Take another breath here.

○ Next, take both hands behind you and place the palms of your hands on your lower back.

○ Close your eyes for the next 2 breaths, adopting the same breath (slowly in through the nose, out through the mouth) and see if you can feel the back of your body moving and expanding into your hands as you breathe.

○ Now take one of your hands to just below your belly button. You should have one hand on the front of your body and the other hand on your lower back. Breathe twice more here, feeling both the back and front of your body while you are breathing.

○ Practise again with your eyes closed. See how you feel. Do you feel calmer, more focused?

ZEN-TEN BREATHE

Simple, quick and effective, this technique will pep up the
energy of a class if the day is starting to take an energetic
nosedive. Keep your arms overhead for the duration of the
exercise. Breathe in and out through the nose, and once
you have practised so that the breath is in unison with the
movements, you can quicken the pace.

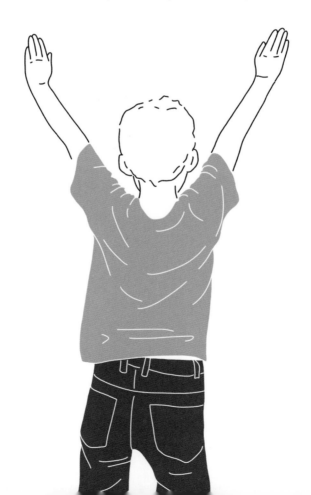

benefits

Peps up energy

Refocuses the mind

Stretches the fingers and hands

○ Take your arms overhead, stretching them up toward the sky. Spread all your fingers wide.

○ Breathe in through the nose, keeping your arms raised. Scrunch your hands into fists.

○ Breathe out through the nose, keeping your arms straight and scrunching your hands into fists.

○ Breathe in, spreading your fingers wide again and letting your hands be "lively".

○ Breathe out, scrunching your hands into fists.

○ Repeat this action until you are comfortable with the breath and hand movements, then you can start to quicken the pace.

○ Repeat 10–20 times.

○ See how you feel. Do you feel a little more energized?

If you have the space, you could create a "breathing room", or dedicated area for breath exercises – at home, at your workplace or at school – where you can take time out to breathe. In the United States, some schools have replaced detention with meditation (of which the foundation is breathwork), with positive results – attendance has increased and suspensions have decreased!

VISUALIZATION

Professional athletes, musicians and business executives use
visualization to improve their performance; and it's important
that we remind our children (and ourselves) of the power of
imagination. Using visualization with breathwork has profound
benefits: we can improve our focus, attention and imagination
and, in the same breath, it reduces stress and tension in the
body and allows us to feel fully relaxed. This is an effective
visualization that children can practise at the end of the day to
help them enjoy a deeper, more peaceful sleep.

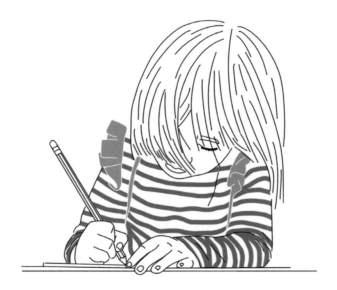

"The true sign of intelligence is not knowledge but imagination."

ALBERT EINSTEIN, GERMAN THEORETICAL PHYSICIST

THE TREE THAT BREATHES

○ Make yourself warm and comfortable. Lie down and place a blanket over your legs and torso.

○ Close your eyes or, if you prefer, close them a little, to allow for a soft gaze. Have your arms at your sides and your feet a little apart, allowing both feet to fall gently out to the side.

○ Allow your body to feel relaxed and notice how it feels on the surface below you. Take a slow, full breath in through the nose and a deep, slow breath out through the mouth. Let your body soften a little further. Now, using your imagination, visualize yourself as a tree. You are the most amazing tree you have ever seen. Imagine your body, belly and legs as the strong trunk, your arms as branches reaching for the sunshine, and your feet as its roots – the foundation and power of this magnificently unique tree. These roots start at the soles of your feet and travel deep into the ground. Breathe in...Breathe out...

○ Wriggle your toes a little and imagine how the mud would feel in between your toes, as the roots travel further and further into the ground. These deep strong roots travel far, and make you feel strong and adventurous.

○ Your legs feel firm and are planted purposefully in the ground.

○ There is only one tree like this in the entire universe. You feel wise. You feel as if you are full of ancient wisdom and you have an important purpose here on the planet.

○ Breathe in slowly... Breathe out through your mouth, listening to the wind-like sound of your breathing.

○ We are all unique magical trees standing in one amazing forest. We are here to help all the other trees grow side-by-side. Let's help each other grow and rise up together.

○ Breathe in slowly... Breathe out through your mouth, listening to the wind-like sound of your breathing.

○ Take a few more breaths here and, when you are ready, gently blink open your eyes; or, if you are feeling sleepy, allow yourself to sleep.

7

THE MUNDANE

"Gratitude can transform common days into thanksgivings, turn routine jobs into joy, and change ordinary opportunities into blessings."

WILLIAM ARTHUR WARD,
AMERICAN WRITER AND COLUMNIST

Sometimes it seems as if we spend a large part of our lives carrying out mundane tasks. We can find ourselves in environments that appear to be a hotbed for feelings of boredom. With all the daily household chores of washing, cleaning and cooking, or being obliged to attend soporific meetings at work – not to mention the hours we spend held up in traffic on the way to and from work, standing in shop queues and catching ourselves staring into space, while we are put on hold for the umpteenth time – at times life can feel lacklustre.

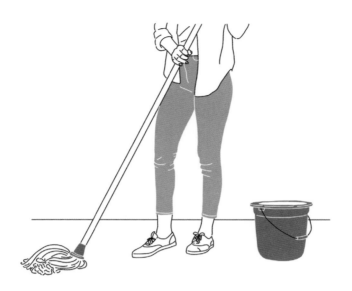

HOW TO TURN MUNDANE MOMENTS INTO A MORE MAGICAL AFFAIR?

Many research studies have revealed that we should actually be embracing these feelings of monotony and tedium. Being bored, if we are patient enough to immerse ourselves fully in it, can be good for us – and can even spark our creativity and productivity.

These days we easily find ourselves filling the pockets of dullness with micro-doses of "mental fidgeting" – checking our phones, a little text here and a short scroll there – leaving very little time for the mind to become fully immersed in those long-lost feelings of "old-fashioned" tedium.

Engaging in breathwork and mindfulness practices can be the perfect antidote to boredom. We spend just over a year of our lives (that's more than six million breaths) engaged in mundane chores, so if we make an effort to connect with our breath and embrace our boredom, then we might find a little magic.

MUNDANE MORNINGS

On average we spend 9 minutes (about 108 breaths) in the shower each morning. Imagine if we used these breaths to energize and start the day feeling 100 per cent alive!

You may already have heard of Wim Hof. He's a bit of a legend in the breathwork world and is often referred to as "The Iceman" – famed for submerging himself in freezing cold water and "brrrreathing". Renowned for breaking records related to cold exposure, his feats include climbing Mount Kilimanjaro in just a pair of shorts, running a half-marathon above the Arctic Circle in his bare feet, and swimming underneath ice for 57.5m (188.6ft).

Personally, when it comes to diving into ice-cold water, I'm more in the "Wimp" Hof category. But I can vouch for the benefits of a quick blast of "cold-water therapy". A trip to Finland introduced me to the sauna-and-cold-shower combination and I have never felt more invigorated. On returning home, I decided to get my "Finnish fix" by immersing myself under daily cold showers.

I have a warm blast first, then at least 2–4 minutes of cold water and it has improved a hundredfold the way I feel. Gone are my seasonal colds; my energy has soared; and I start the day feeling very "alive". Give it a go with this breath exercise.

benefits of a cold shower

Increases a sense of alertness

Boosts the circulation

Improves the immune system

Eases stress

Relieves depression

Can be the ultimate "wake-up" call

O Following a pleasant warm shower, be brave and turn the tap to the coldest setting.

O "Brrrr"eathe... Draw the breath in through the nose.

O Open your mouth wide, really feeling the muscles in your face stretch, and breathe out through the mouth with one whispered "Oooo" sound.

O Breathe in again through the nose, feeling the cold water on your skin. Notice which parts of your body are most sensitive to the cold. The upper chest, belly or back?

O Open your mouth wide and make a whispered "Ahhhhhh".

O Repeat for 5–10 cycles, with an "Oooo" then "Ahhh", then allow the breath to return to its natural pace.

O Notice how you are feeling. Refreshed? More awake?

O Start with a minute, building up to 2–5 minutes on the cold setting.

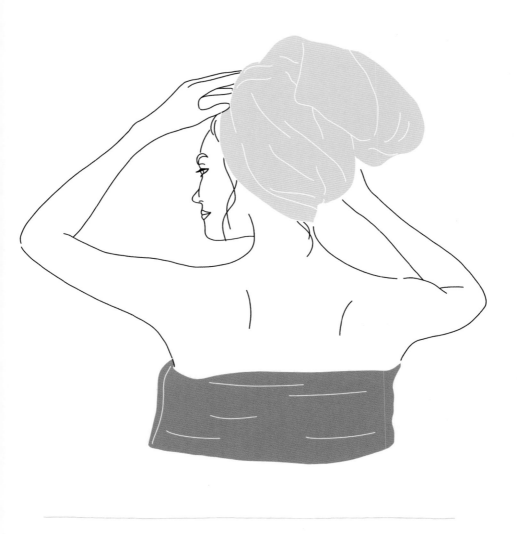

If this sounds way too intense, start by splashing your face with cold water and then, over a week or two, build some resilience and choose a body part that will get a cold blast, until you are eventually fully immersed. Before you know it, you will feel amazing and won't be able to shower without a cold-water finale.

KNOCK YOUR SOCKS OFF

It's easy to weave a little yoga and conscious breathing into your daily routine. If you tack an exercise onto a morning activity (getting dressed/cleaning/picking things up from the floor), you will soon develop a healthy habit. Next time you bend down to slip on your socks or shoes, think "Breathe".

Allow yourself 5–10 breaths in this calming yoga pose: Uttanasana, or Forward Bending Pose, is ideal to practise just before popping on (or picking up) your socks.

○ Position your legs hip-width apart, hands on your hips. Slowly roll your torso down, bending from the hips.

○ Allow your head, arms and hands to hang down toward the floor. Make sure there is no tension in the neck muscles.

○ Be sure your face, arms, head and hands are all relaxed. Allow yourself to feel floppy.

○ Let your fingertips dangle toward the floor and "hang" here for a few breaths.

○ Breathe in through the nose, out through the nose. Allow the tip of your tongue to rest on the roof of your mouth.

○ Feel the back and front of your body move with each breath.

○ Take 3 long and slow breaths (for beginners) and build up to 10 breaths over time. Don't stay in this position longer than a minute. With each exhalation, notice if the hands reach a little closer to the floor.

○ If you have more time on your hands, scientists recommend that you try to touch your toes at least 30 times a day to improve flexibility. (It really works!)

b e n e f i t s

Rejuvenates the mind and relaxes the nervous system

Stretches the hips, hamstrings and calves

Builds strength in the thighs and knees

Boosts direct blood flow to the head

Activates the abdominal muscles

Increases flexibility of the spine

Stimulates the kidneys, liver and spleen, thus
bringing about a sense of physical relief

Improves the digestion

Reduces high blood pressure

Can play a major role in treating the symptoms of
several conditions, including the menopause, asthma,
headaches and insomnia

Alleviates symptoms of stress, anxiety, mild
depression and fatigue of the body and mind

Widely considered therapeutic for infertility,
osteoporosis and sinusitis

NB: Refrain from practising this pose if you have any chronic conditions, or if you
have a history of any injury in your knee joints, ankle joints or back.

QUEUE-BREATHE

I created this "breathing game" a few years ago, while stuck
in a seemingly endless queue for passport control at an
airport. My view was a vast sea of heads, with a sense of
tired frustration in the air. With two young children in tow,
I wondered how I was going to remain calm and uplifted with
such an arduous wait in prospect.

Inspired by breathwork, and looking for the positives,
I took a few deep breaths, scanning the scene before me
for something beautiful. Then I took two slow breaths
and moved on in search of another moment of loveliness,
choosing anything in the long line of people – something as
simple as a brightly coloured jacket, the smile on someone's
face while talking to a loved one, other people's children
playing or the elderly couple holding hands. I found it
incredible how much beauty there was around me. This
worked so well for me that it's now a breathing game that
I often play on the train to work or while queuing in a shop.
When you transform the mundane into a mindful moment,
there's always some form of beauty nearby.

"The cure for boredom is curiosity. There is no cure for curiosity."

ELLEN PARR

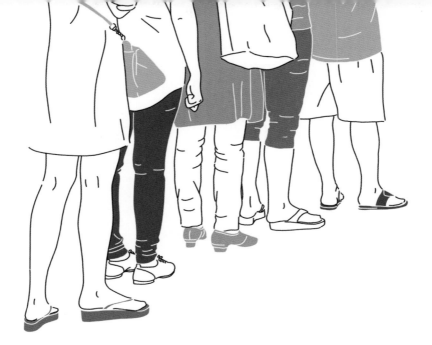

benefits

Transports you from "boredom to beauty"

Brings you into the present moment

Cultivates gratitude

Brings a mindful practice into your day

O Breathe...in. Scan your immediate environment for a beautiful colour, moment or scene.

O Repeat a few times until you are in a more positive frame of mind.

O Breathe out while holding your gaze here.

TRAFFIC-JAM BREATHE

When you are faced with the slowest Internet connection, or are put on hold for eternity, or are stuck in an endless traffic jam on a hot day, here's a cooling exercise to help you release the frustration and pent-up anger. It works in just a few minutes.

Sitali is a classic yoga breathing technique, often translated as "the cooling breath", because it is said to have a cooling and calming effect on the nervous system. To practise Sitali, ideally you need to be able to curl the sides of your tongue inward into a U-shape.

○ Sit in a comfortable position with your head, neck and spine in alignment.

○ Take a few full diaphragmatic breaths for a few minutes, then open your mouth and form the lips into an O-shape.

○ If you can, curl your tongue lengthwise and gently poke it out of your mouth. (If you can't roll your tongue, place the underside of your tongue to the roof of your mouth).

○ Breathe, sipping the air in through your tongue and into your mouth. Focus your attention on the cooling sensation of the breath as your abdomen and lower ribs expand.

○ Draw your tongue back into the mouth, exhaling through the nostrils.

○ Repeat for 2–3 minutes. Then return to nasal breathing for a minute, and repeat the cooling breath for another couple of minutes.

SMILE BREATHE

Bring a splash of brightness into any tedious moment with a simple smile. However you are feeling right now, try and smile. This small, effortless upturn of the lips sends so many feel-good vibes to your brain that can benefit your health and happiness.

benefits

Activates the release of neuropeptides (signalling molecules), the mood-boosting neurotransmitters dopamine and serotonin, and endorphins (feel-good chemicals)

Helps the body to relax

Lowers the heart rate

O Soften your face and shoulders.

O Breathe...in through the nose.

O Smile with your lips closed.

O Breathe out through the nose.

O Smile.

O Keep the breath and face relaxed.

O Notice how you feel. A little lighter? A sprinkling of happiness?

"Sometimes your joy is the source of your smile, but sometimes your smile can be the source of your joy."

THICH NHAT HANH, VIETNAMESE BUDDHIST MONK

"BORED BUDDHA" BREATHE

Boredom can often happen when we are in a situation over which we have little control. But we always have the opportunity to control our breathing. If you can find a way to embrace boredom, then you may surprise yourself by having a brilliant idea or a flash of inspiration.

Using this time to reconnect with your breath will enable you to build a steady breathwork practice into your days. Connecting with these moments of boredom in a more positive way can enable you to feel inspired and energized.

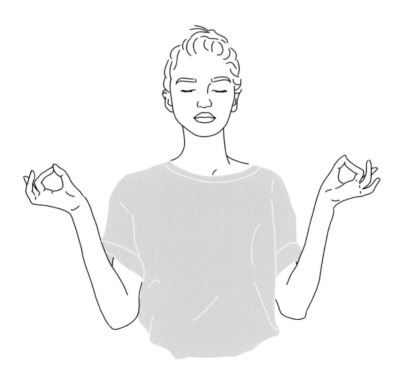

benefits

Has a positive effect on the brain's limbic system, which is responsible for good moods

○ Adopt a comfortable seated position.

○ Place the thumb of the right hand on the pad of your middle finger. Apply light pressure here.

○ Repeat with the left hand, so that both hands mirror this mudra or hand position.

○ Raise the chin slightly and, with closed eyes if this is comfortable, direct your eye gaze upward to the centre of your forehead.

○ Curl the tip of the tongue toward the back of the roof of your mouth, so that the underside of your tongue presses on the roof.

It will feel as if your tongue is folded in half.

○ Breathe... Simply observe the four stages of breathing (inhale/ the pause/exhale/the pause) while applying pressure between the middle fingers and thumbs.

○ Slow the entire breath process down. Let the mind wander, but focus on the breath. Do you feel any sensations between the thumbs and middle fingers? Any feelings on the roof of the mouth, the tongue or the face?

○ If the mind wanders off again, simply bring it back to the rhythm of your breath.

8

CLEAN AIR

"For most of us plants are just a decorative element, something aesthetic, but they are also something else."

FEDERICO BRILLI, ITALIAN PLANT PHYSIOLOGIST

Indoor air pollution can be traced back to prehistoric times, when humans first moved to milder climates and it became necessary to construct shelters and use fire inside their caves for cooking, warmth and light. Fire led to exposure to high levels of pollution, as evidenced by the soot that has been found in various prehistoric caves.

From the modest cave to today's modern homes and offices, it seems we have become accustomed to the indoor way of life, with the majority of us finding that we spend a large proportion of our lives indoors. A revealing report by the US Environmental Protection Agency concluded that people living in industrialized countries spend as much of 90 per cent of their time inside.

Indoor air pollution is ranked as one of the world's greatest public-health risks, so much so that there is even a particular condition related to it. Sick Building Syndrome, or SBS, occurs when your living space or workplace is compromised by a long list of adverse conditions, such as poor ventilation, dusty rooms, chemical-infused air, high humidity and inadequate lighting, to name but a few. The combination of these conditions puts many people's health at risk.

With an increase in the number of pupils, employees, residents and patients being affected by SBS, there are growing reports of symptoms related to this modern-day disease. Escalating complaints of breathing difficulties, runny noses, sneezing, headaches, throat irritation and poor concentration are an indicator, perhaps, that it's high time we looked seriously at improving the quality of the indoor air we breathe.

Given the rising number of people living and working in environments with sub-standard air quality, it comes as no surprise that there is a boom in the popularity of air-purifying houseplants. Fortunately, nature loves equilibrium and, according to the theory of biophilia (humans' innate need to connect to the natural world, see page 106), we can help to improve our indoor air quality. Are a few pots of green foliage really enough to clean the air we breathe? NASA thinks so...

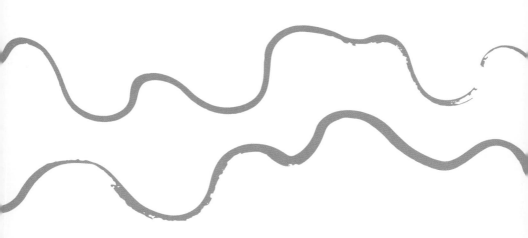

AIR-PURIFYING INDOOR PLANTS

In 1989 NASA conducted a study into the air-purifying qualities of indoor plants and discovered seven super-plants, which were particularly efficient at absorbing the most harmful chemicals found in indoor air. While other plants in the study were absorbing one or two of these invisible killers, the super-plants were absorbing all of the most harmful volatile organic compounds (VOCs) tested. These plants were sucking up the by-products of vehicle exhaust fumes – which can creep insidiously into our work and home environments – and of cleaning products, such as the carcinogenic benzene, formaldehyde, xylene and toluene, efficiently purifying the air and instantly creating a healthier breathing space.

Because the NASA study was conducted in a highly controlled environment, it is hard to conclude exactly how many pot plants we need in order to enjoy breathing in clean air in our immediate environment. However, with the knowledge that green spaces can have a positive effect on our general health, I would suggest creating a plant oasis in every room of your home and office, with as many of the following super-plants as your space and budget permit.

"There are air-purifying plants, and then there are Super Plants."

SEVEN SUPER-PLANTS

These super-plants topped NASA's list for their air-purifying qualities, and removed all four of the most harmful VOCs found in our indoor air. Surround yourself with these super-plants and you will be breathing cleaner air, while welcoming a corner of calm into your work and living space.

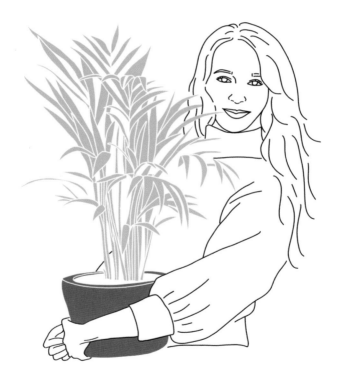

NB: Some indoor plants are toxic to dogs and cats.

1

SNAKE PLANT
(*Sansevieria trifasciata var. laurentii*)

Also, rather amusingly, called "Mother-in-Law's Tongue". Whereas most other plants release carbon dioxide at night (in the absence of photosynthesis), the *Sansevieria* continues to produce oxygen. Have a few in the bedroom to boost your lung health while you are sleeping.

2

PEACE LILY
(*Spathiphyllum spp.*)

Perhaps the prettiest air filter you will find, the peace lily topped NASA's list for improving air quality. It likes moderate light and high humidity, so keep it away from cold, draughty windows. Keep the soil moist, but be careful not to overwater it.

3

BAMBOO PALM
(*Chamaedorea seifrizii*)

Native to Mexico and Central America, this dwarf plant doesn't grow taller than 1.5m (5ft). It loves light and humidity, will filter your home or office of benzene and trichloroethylene. It is easy to keep and will brighten up any desk space.

4

RED-EDGED DRACAENA
(*Dracaena marginata*)

The "dragon tree" is grown for its dramatic foliage and carefree nature. Make sure you look for purple-red edges on ribbon-like leaves, because there are many species of dracaena.

5

ENGLISH IVY
(*Hedera helix*)

This ivy is one of the great all-round air purifiers and is easy company to keep. It loves a lot of light and not too much water, as it likes being kept on the dry side.

6

SPIDER PLANT
(*Chlorophytum comosum*)

This plant likes to absorb various harmful compounds. Spider plants are very easy to grow, prefer dry soil and thrive in cooler homes. Keep them away from direct sunlight, which can burn the leaves. Pop them somewhere with bright to moderate light.

7

FLORIST'S CHRYSANTHEMUM
(*Chrysanthemum morifolium*)

Regular watering is crucial. Keep chrysanthemum plants where they can receive good air circulation, and avoid excess humidity.

OUTDOOR AIR POLLUTION

While learning to improve the way we breathe can have a positive effect on our health and happiness, worryingly, air pollution has become one of the biggest public-health crises of our time. Poor air quality is now being linked to many diseases, from respiratory illnesses and stunted lung growth, to cancer, heart disease, dementia and even mental-health issues in teenagers. It can also contribute to miscarriage and low birth weight. In the UK, air pollution is estimated to cut short 36,000 lives a year (including those of 9,500 Londoners).

Fortunately, some inspirational groups are raising awareness of this global crisis. Here's what Jemima Hartshorn, co-founder of Mums for Lungs — a London-based network of parents campaigning for cleaner air — has to say:

"The World Health Organization estimates that annually 7 million lives are cut short as a result of ambient air pollution. The most common elements of air pollution are NO_2 (a gas) and particulate matter (PM2.5, P10). When breathing high levels of NO_2 and PM on a regular basis the lining of the lung inflames, and the tiny particulates can enter our blood streams and thereby our organs, including the brain, as they are too small to be filtered by the lungs."

There is hope, though: in the light of evidence of the consequences for our health and with technological improvements, vehicles are becoming cleaner and cars that use fossil fuel are falling out of favour with governments and cities across the world. Some cities are even implementing regular car-free days.

HOW TO IMPROVE THE AIR WE BREATHE

We can do a lot to reduce air pollution, as well as limiting our exposure to it on a daily basis. Mums for Lungs suggests the following ways in which we can improve the air we breathe:

1

Most importantly, we need fewer miles driven across our roads. Reconsider every car trip you plan to take, and reduce your home deliveries. Can you pick up a parcel in a shop nearby, to reduce the miles driven by the delivery van (and reduce the fumes in your road)? Is there a bus to your destination? Can you combine two trips you need to take?

 4

Lobby your government to phase out diesel engines as soon as possible, and support your city in significantly restricting the use of road vehicles (clean-air zones). Public transport needs to be better, cheaper and more accessible. Walking across the countryside and any city or village should be a pleasure.

 2

If you are replacing your car, can you buy one with lower emissions? Perhaps even an electric vehicle? Perhaps you can even make do using carshare?

 5

Tell other people about air pollution, so that they can reduce their own emissions and protect themselves and their loved ones. Thank you!

 3

To protect yourself from pollution, walk on back streets and stay as far as possible from the kerb. Pollution is lower the further away you are from transport vehicles. (By the way, pollution is generally higher inside a car....)

 6

And lastly, most sources of air pollution are also major contributors to the climate crisis. So by reducing air pollution we also reduce our carbon footprint and contribute to a healthier planet.

9

RELATIONSHIPS

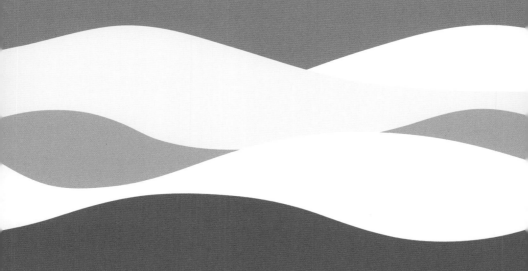

"And now here is my secret, a very simple secret:
It is only with the heart that one can see rightly;
what is essential is invisible to the eye."

ANTOINE DE SAINT-EXUPÉRY, FRENCH AUTHOR AND POET

Every encounter in life can stir certain feelings within us – a slow internet connection can result in a flash of frustration, completing a new solo project can leave you with a sense of relief, reading a good novel can make you laugh or cry and you can feel vulnerable when visiting new places alone. You can be in your own company and experience a sea of feelings. However, it's often in our personal relationships, when our deeper, stronger emotions are triggered, shaken and stirred.

The word "emotion" derives from the Latin "emotus" ("emouvoir" in French), which means to stir up or move out. Emotional energy is born to move; e-motion is purely "energy in motion".

If you feel an emotion in the body, for example, when you have just received some sad news, you may feel a lump in the throat, tears may start to well up, and if you don't feel comfortable fully expressing this with a good cry, you tend to hold your breath. This instantly halts the movement of two natural healing processes. So, where do these held-back tears go?

Regular contraction of the respiratory muscles (when suppressing feelings and the breath) can create a build-up of unnecessary tension throughout the body. We literally store our emotions in our muscles and tissues: words can get "stuck in our throat"; we can keep a "stiff upper lip", we need to "get things out of our system"; "gut feelings" are sometimes ignored; we can have a "heavy heart", or have to deal with people who are "a pain in the neck" (or the backside!); we get "knots in our stomach" and we carry "the weight of the world on our shoulders".

These bottled-up emotions can eventually morph into physical discomfort, having a detrimental effect on how we feel – mentally, physically and emotionally. Just as we have forgotten how to breathe well, we have also lost the innate ability to heal well, too.

Sometimes life throws us more challenging moments for our body and mind to cope with and we don't feel like we can breathe at all; we suddenly lose people we love, people we trust betray us, our home or country suddenly becomes divided, or we are forced to split from those we hold dear. From divorce to war, we can find ourselves in new places with new people, trying to navigate our way through new internal and external landscapes simultaneously.

Other times, more traumatic experiences can make us "freeze" and we feel nothing at all, and numbness prevails. Breathwork, talking and movement-based therapies can serve us positively during these moments in life when we don't feel like moving at all.

Integrating these emotions, whereby we acknowledge and accept them, breathe with them, and release them, can help us to feel lighter and less burdened. Only then can we start to feel alive and ready to build and engage in healthy relationships again.

Stacy Matulis is a Somatic and Depth Psychologist and breath worker, who works with couples and runs a private Somatic Healing and Coaching practice in South Pasadena, California. Here she offers us some sound advice, using breath awareness, to help us navigate our way through challenging times.

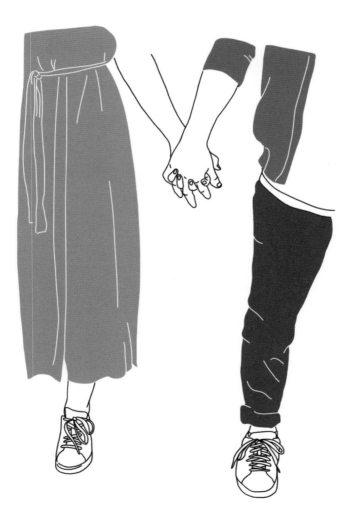

THE RESILIENT ZONE

In any intimate relationship, "missing" one another is an easy thing to do.

"Mis"-understandings, "mis"-interpretations, arguments, projections and/or past traumas can all affect a person in a way that makes it difficult to fully hear the other person.

In psychology there is a place called the "resilient zone". This is the place where you feel calm in your body, you have clarity of thought and your nervous system feels regulated.

When a person is taken out of this resilient zone, their blood pressure and heart rate rises, their breath becomes quick and shallow, and their body goes into "fight or flight" mode. When operating from this place of fear, we habitually defend our territory and promptly put up defensive barriers in order to protect ourselves. It becomes almost impossible to be receptive and is a challenge not to be reactive.

So many relationships suffer because their disagreements turn into fights, where one or both partners fall out of their resilient zone and neither feels fully heard.

One way to change this reaction is to begin to learn and experience, with awareness, what it feels like to leave your resilient zone, by tracking the felt experience in your body. Upon recognizing that you have become shut down, you can notice that you are in a safe place, you do not need to physically defend yourself and begin to breathe long, deep breaths to return to a calm and present state.

Stacy Matulis coaches couples to "track" this for themselves. If one (or both) has entered this defensive state, they make an agreement to say: "Let's go back to zero". What this means is, let's drop into a breath practice so we have a chance of hearing one another from a calmer space. It's important that both partners agree to drop into the breath practice when either partner says "Let's go back to zero", so it doesn't become a blame game of who is or is not in the resilient zone!

So, in a partnership, when a moment arrives that one or both of you fall into a defensive state, you can practise a simple breathing ritual to engender calmer communication. Both of you should take 5–15 long, slow, deep and quiet breaths (in through the nose, out through the mouth) to bring yourselves back into the "resilient zone". From this place, track your feelings, soften your heart, look into each other's eyes to reconnect, and try to start communicating again.

The practice of "going back to zero" with the full conscious breath ritual gives both partners a chance to refresh, drop their defences, and get back into a centred place and be able to discuss matters with more clarity of mind.

BUILDING RESILIENCE

Building a daily breath practice can increase your emotional strength as by regularly stimulating the parasympathetic nervous system you will naturally be able to spend more time in your resilient zone. Commit to practising the following breath technique for 5–10 minutes every morning for a week (or two!) and notice if you begin to react differently to any challenging scenarios that arise.

ALTERNATE NOSTRIL BREATHING

This ancient yogic breath technique is still popular today and is practised by CEOs, politicians, athletes and executives to help them manage stress and anxiety. This simple yet effective exercise is best practised in the morning so you can start your day in a calmer, more resilient state of mind.

benefits

Builds emotional resilience

Soothes the nervous system

Regulates body temperature

Balances left and right sides of brain

Increases lung volume

Reduces blood pressure and heart rate

- Sit in an upright, relaxed position.

- Take a few long slow breaths, in and out through the nose: when you breathe in feel your belly rise, and your sitting bones connect with the floor or chair. When you breathe out, soften your shoulders, face and jaw. Always allow space between your top and bottom jaw. Relax your hands and face. Over-thinking a situation can make the facial muscles tense – encourage these muscles to soften.

- Scan your body for any tension or emotions. Are there feelings in your heart? The pit of your stomach? Jaw or head? Or maybe there is an overall numbness? Recognize if there is any energy in motion in the body.

- Raise your right hand to your face and using your index or ring finger, press on the outside of your LEFT nostril, enough to block 90 per cent of the airflow.

- Inhale slowly through your RIGHT nostril. Visualize the air entering your body as a light colour.

- Hold the breath in momentarily, bringing your awareness to the expanse of the lower belly.

- With the right thumb, block the RIGHT nostril and breathe out slowly through the LEFT nostril. Visualize the air leaving your body as a dark colour. Allow the exhale to be longer than the inhale.

- Now breathe in through the LEFT nostril, hold the breath and (release the thumb) breathe out through RIGHT nostril.

- Then breathe in through the RIGHT nostril. Suspend the breath. breathe out through the LEFT nostril. Repeat this rhythm for 5–10 rounds.

- For the final round, take a few breaths through both nostrils.

- Notice if any of these feelings are lighter or if this energy starts to move you may notice ripples of energy throughout the body.

SUPPRESSED EMOTIONS

There are also specific breath exercises for releasing those feelings we suppress the most, namely sadness, grief, anger, fear and love.

I was first introduced to the following yoga breath techniques by a wonderful teacher called Stan Cortes, with whom I enjoyed a year-long Hatha yoga teacher training. His beautifully curated classes, focusing on how to connect with and release energy from the body, always helped me shift heavier energy in a gentle and safe way. I left his classes feeling emotionally lighter and more connected to the world and to those around me.

Stan has been teaching Kundalini Yoga for over 26 years. When it comes to the adage: "you have to feel it to heal it", these particular breath techniques he teaches are strikingly effective. Time is the greatest healer, but only if we use some of this time to heal. Give yourself permission to connect with your breath and fully immerse yourself in each of these breath exercises.

CALM HEART BREATH MEDITATION

When the heart is heavy or you are feeling sad, this breath meditation can re-balance your energies and relieve any pain. Give yourself 5–15 minutes to practise this breath meditation, allow any feelings to be felt and, if tears come, breathe deeply and let them go.

benefits

Relieves anxiety

Stills the heart

Strengthens the heart and lungs

Shifts your perception of a relationship

Releases sadness and heavy emotions

Brings awareness to an upper chest breath

POSTURE: Sit in a comfortable position, with a tall spine and the tip of your tongue to the roof of your mouth (for well-practised yogis use Jalandhara Bandha/chin lock). If there is a particular relationship you wish to work on, you can bring that person to mind during this exercise.

POSITION OF THE HANDS:

Left hand: Place the left palm on the centre of the chest at the heart centre, as shown. Your palm should be flat against your chest and your fingers together and pointing to the right. The centre of the chest is the natural home of prana (life force) and creates a deep stillness at this point.

Right hand: Bring the tip of your thumb to touch the tip of your index finger. Raise your right hand up to your right side. Your elbow is relaxed near your side with your forearm perpendicular to the ground. Your palm faces forward, your three remaining fingers point up. (Tip: your fingers should look like they are mimicking the "OK" sign.) Your right hand is placed in this position to bring you into action and analysis, and your left hand is placed in a receptive, relaxed mudra in the position of peace.

EYES: Either close your eyes or look straight ahead with your eyes slightly closed.

O Inhale slowly and deeply through both nostrils. Then suspend the breath in and slightly lift your chest. Retain the breath in for as long as is comfortable.

O Then exhale through the nose smoothly, gradually and completely.

O When you have exhaled, hold the breath out for as long as you can without discomfort. Release the breath if you feel any contractions in the diaphragm or intercostal muscles.

O Concentrate on the flow of the breath. Notice what happens in each part of this breath technique. The inhale. The hold. The exhale. The hold.

O Practise for no longer than 15 minutes. Each breath round should bring a new sense of lightness to the body.

FINISH: Inhale and exhale fully for a minute with no pauses.

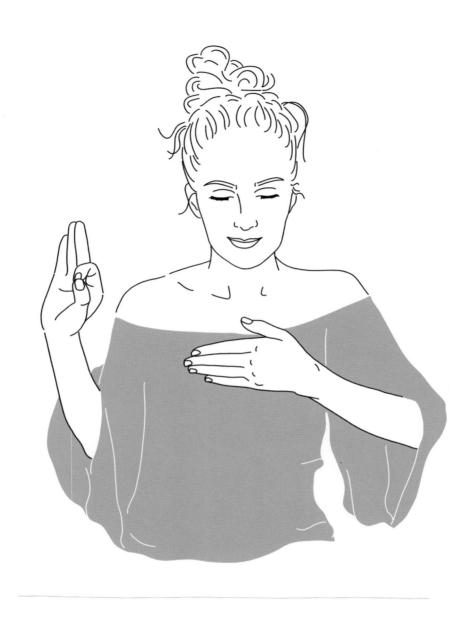

"*Happiness is the absence of the striving for happiness.*"

CHUANG TZU, CHINESE PHILOSOPHER

RECONNECT BREATH

Stan Cortes says: "I used this breathing technique a lot when I became a father. The transition from being an individual to a parent is profound and this breath technique is extremely valuable for those moments when you start to lose reference of who you are. This helped me reconnect with my wife, my newborn daughter and myself. "

benefits

Calms and releases fear

Gives you a sense of focus and openness

Brings your brain and heart to a coherent state

Balances the nervous system

For beginners, start with a slow count between 5 and 10 (for each part) and over time build up to the maximum count of 15.

POSTURE: Sit in a comfortable position with a tall spine. Your chin should be parallel to the floor and the tip of the tongue touching the roof of your mouth. Allow space between your top and bottom teeth.

- Inhale through your nose for a count of 15.

- Hold the breath in for a count of 15, have a sense of "lift" in the spine, and relax your shoulders.

- Exhale for a slow count of 15.

- Repeat a few times.

(8 STROKE) FIND PEACE BREATHE

This can be practised to help you to overcome any resentment, anger or frustration. You will notice an energetic shift in just a few rounds, but if you have the time, set aside 11 minutes for this exercise to experience its full transformational effects.

benefits

Releases pent-up anger

Calms the nervous system

Releases energy and stress

Relaxes the mind

Transforms negative feelings

POSTURE: Sit with your spine straight, chin parallel to the floor, and gently draw the shoulder blades together so the chest has a slight lift. Keep your eyes closed.

O Inhale for 8 strokes through the nose.

O Exhale fully through the nose in one long, deep, powerful breath.

O Repeat for up to 11 minutes.

FINISH:

O Inhale deeply, hold the breath for 5–10 counts, and exhale.

O Inhale deeply, hold the breath for 10–20 counts and roll your shoulders. Exhale powerfully.

O Inhale deeply, hold the breath for 10–20 counts and roll your shoulders as fast as you can. Exhale and relax.

LOVE & MAGIC BREATHE

One of the most surprising and charming discoveries from my years of teaching breathwork is the amount of positive emotions we suppress, too. How best to connect with these layers of suppressed love? It's simple, and the best medicine of all – laughter. Practise this exercise every day for a week and see if your general mood shifts. (Do avoid if you have a hernia.)

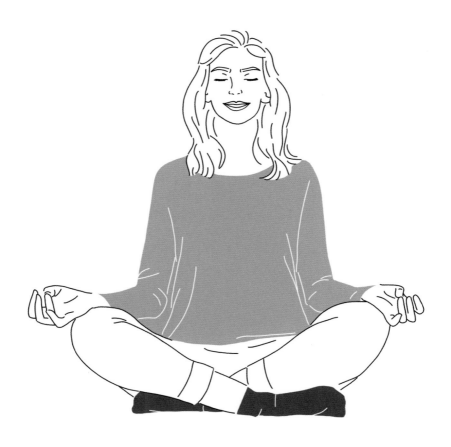

b e n e f i t s

Lowers blood pressure

Reduces stress hormones

Releases endorphins

Works your core muscles

O This exercise is best experienced lying down to free the diaphragm.

O Breathing out through the mouth, sound the words "Ha ha ha ha" until the breath runs out.

O Inhale deeply through the nose. Smile.

O On the exhale quicken and change the pitch of the "Hahahahahahahahaha" sounds until a real laugh forms.

O Inhale deeply though the nose and smile.

O Repeat for a few rounds (for no more than 2 minutes). Allow the real laughs to come and go.

O End with a few deep breaths, a full heart and a sweet smile.

"We are all here for a spell. Get all the good laughs you can."

WILL ROGERS, AMERICAN ACTOR

10

EATING & EXERCISE

"You are what you eat eats."

MICHAEL POLLAN, AMERICAN AUTHOR

OXYGEN + FOOD = ENERGY

The oxygen we breathe is produced by some form of green plant life, with the majority being produced from the life-giving (and extremely beautiful) diatoms. This incredible, microscopic single cell algae, has light absorbing molecules (chlorophylls) that collect light energy from the sun and converts it into chemical energy through photosynthesis.

As diatoms remove carbon-dioxide from the atmosphere, the CO_2 is converted to organic carbon in the form of sugar, and oxygen is released – ready for us to inhale.

This oxygen is absorbed into the lungs when we breathe in (external respiration) as the carbon dioxide is removed (gas exchange). The oxygen is then passed into the blood stream (internal respiration) and travels to each one of our 37 trillion cells. Each aerobic (those which need oxygen) cell will absorb this oxygen (cellular respiration) to enable it to produce energy, with the help of the food we eat.

We can survive without food for over a month, without water for around 3 days but can only survive without oxygen for about 3 minutes. It goes without saying, breathing is number one when it comes to our survival, but when it comes to feeling full of natural energy, the food we eat and water we drink are vital components to feeling well.

"THE THIRD LUNG"

Here, Sybille Gebhardt, naturopath and yoga teacher, shares her knowledge of certain foods that can support the health and functioning of the respiratory system.

"In Chinese medicine, the skin is referred to as 'the third lung'. The skin breathes and eliminates toxic waste just as the lungs do. The condition of our skin can sometimes be an indicator of the health of our respiratory system. For instance, skin problems such as eczema, psoriasis and rashes can be associated with imbalances in the body that also relate to the lungs.

We can keep this 'third lung' healthy through skin brushing, hot and cold showers, using products made with non-harmful ingredients and most importantly, eating healthy, organic, local and seasonal vegetables, fresh fruits, whole grains, seeds, nuts, fermented foods and fresh oily cold-water fish.

Your gastrointestinal tract is lined with a hundred million nerve cells and the function of these neurons – and the production of neurotransmitters like serotonin – is highly influenced by the billions of 'good' bacteria that make up your intestinal microbiome. Your gastrointestinal tract produces 95 per cent of the chemical serotonin, which helps to regulate sleep, appetite and manage your moods.

These foods will help the complex and diverse microbiome of bacteria that live in your intestines, on your skin, inside your mouth, and in many other areas of your body, which are essential to your health and happiness. It is also important to identify and eliminate food allergens or sensitivities and, if necessary, follow a hypoallergenic diet.

Generally, dairy products, wheat and sugar are considered 'mucus causing' foods or those which can cause inflammation in the body (depleting the functioning of the respiratory system) and should be eliminated during stressful times or acute infection of the airways, even if you are not intolerant to these foods.

The same foods, eaten by some people, can affect the body and mind in many ways. For instance, one person may eat a bowl of porridge and feel satisfied and energized, but another may be left feeling bloated, tired and heavy. Bringing your awareness to how you feel after eating certain foods can steer you towards making healthier choices – and you will start eating more of those foods that leave you feeling light and energized.

A healthy respiratory system and glowing skin also needs plenty of fluids. The amount varies slightly depending on body size, air temperature and humidity, as well as how much you sweat, or if you are ill. The ideal water intake is around 2 litres (3½ pints) per day (in some countries, tap water is highly chlorinated and it's best to avoid this, as chlorine can irritate the lungs and skin). Fluids can also be taken in the form of herbal teas, soups, stews and swollen foods (those which need water for soaking or cooking) such as short grain brown rice, nuts and seeds."

HOMEMADE SMOOTHIES
FOR HEALTHY LUNGS

With our fast-paced lives, smoothies are a convenient way to consume highly nutritious foods as part of a well-balanced diet. Quick and easy to make, and a great way to boost your lung health, here are a selection of ingredients you can pick and mix to make a healthy breakfast which is a great way (for the gut and lungs) to start the day. Add one ingredient from each layer, blend, drink and take a deeper, fuller breath!

CHOOSE ONE INGREDIENT FROM EACH LAYER.
MIX AND DRINK.

LIQUID LAYER	LUNG CLEANSER (FRUIT)	LUNG BOOSTER	LUNG PROTECTOR
Rice milk	Acai berry	Almond or pumpkin seed butter	Fresh ginger
Almond milk	Apricot	Pre-soaked walnuts	Fresh turmeric
Oat milk	Peach	Vegan protein	root (or powder
Coconut water	Blueberries	powders	if you can't get
Coconut kefir	Dark seedless	Maca root	fresh root)
Purified water	grapes	Ground flaxseeds	Cinnamon
	Dark cherries	Aloe vera juice	Raw cacao
	Raspberries	1 shot of coffee	powder
	Avocado	(good for asthmatics)	Matcha green tea
	Pomegranate	Kale, parsley or	powder
		spinach	
		Bee pollen	

LUNG PROTECTOR

LUNG BOOSTER

LUNG CLEANSER
(FRUIT)

LIQUID LAYER

"Let food be thy medicine and medicine be thy food."

HIPPOCRATES, ANCIENT GREEK PHYSICIAN

BREATHE...

The manner in which we eat our food is also worth considering. Practising a few breath-focused techniques can encourage you to eat more mindfully, and relaxation plays a critical role in how well we digest our food.

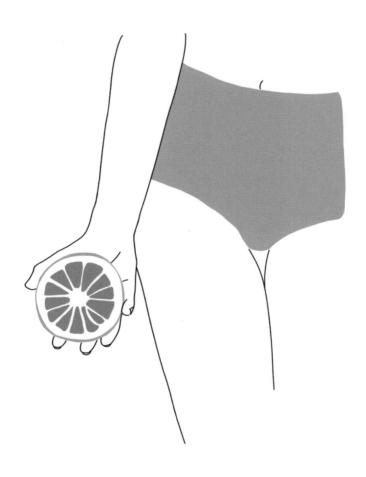

benefits

Calms the nervous system

Brings you into the present moment

Reduces stress hormones, which
can affect your blood sugar

Makes you less likely to eat sugary foods

Aids digestion

Can prevent over-eating

STARTER:

Take 3–5 deep breaths before you eat. This will shift your nervous system
into a "rest-and-digest" state and this more relaxed mood will allow your
digestive system to extract the maximum nutrition from your food.

MAIN:

Take 2–3 breaths in between mouthfuls. Pay special attention to the
textures, flavours and aromas of your food.

DESSERT:

Before you reach for dessert, take a few slow, mindful breaths and notice
if you are full...or maybe you do have room for cheesecake!

EXERCISE

Russell Storey is a breathworker and senior trainer with the Transformational Breath® Foundation. His name is apt, for he has an inspirational story to share:

"After using the power of breathwork to recover from a severe burnout experience, I felt a new bout of energy and set a simple goal to become stronger and fitter.

With the support of work colleagues, I began to run for 20 minutes at lunchtimes and gradually built up the confidence (and stamina) to run a weekly 5km parkrun. Over the next few years, I completed a number of 10km runs, half marathons, and triathlons. In 2018, I completed two 70.3 Ironman Triathlons."

Here he shares his thoughts and his "go-to" breath technique for building awareness, strength and stamina:

"Whether you're a weekend walker or a serious competitive athlete, the health benefits of regular exercise are widely known.

Moving your body in a healthy way is good for you and as anyone who exercises regularly will tell you having an active body is not just about physical health but is also the cornerstone of mental and emotional health too.

In these increasingly complex and stress-inducing times, getting back to basics and accelerating your heart rate for 15 minutes a day can have significant benefits for your wellbeing. Short spurts of vigorous exercise allow more blood and oxygen to get to our cells and help all our organs function to their optimum levels."

THE FROG

Many athletes use breathing techniques to calm their nerves before a sporting event and to boost the overall efficiency of their respiratory system. But some can over-breathe and while certain breath techniques can help to stabilize their breath pattern, only a select few breath exercises can help boost the cardiovascular system. The "Frog" is by far the best.

If you haven't got time for a run or a swim, this technique is very effective for building cardiovascular fitness and is one of the few breath exercises that can increase oxygen supply to the muscles. It's quick and easy to practice but there are a few precautions – if you have any knee or ankle issues, take it easy, and start with a few repetitions. Stop any time you feel any discomfort or dizziness.

benefits

Helps your circulation

Boosts the cardiovascular system

Increases oxygen saturation

Builds stamina

"How art thou out of breath when thou hast breath
To say to me that thou art out of breath?"

WILLIAM SHAKESPEAPE, ENGLISH POET AND PLAYWRIGHT

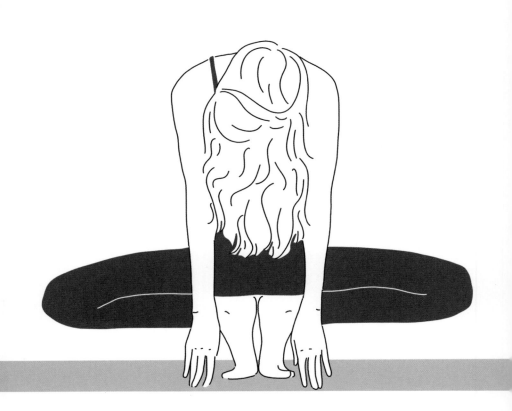

- **POSTURE:** Place your feet apart with your heels touching (come up on to your toes if you can) and balance yourself in a squat position, legs bent, knees pointing outward and bottom toward the floor. Keep your arms straight (to the inside of your legs) with your fingertips touching the floor to help you balance. Keep your eyes open.

- Exhale through the nose and straighten your legs. If you can, try keeping your fingertips on the floor (if you cannot straighten your legs totally, keep them bent and keep your fingertips on the floor). Try to bring your nose as close as possible to your knees. While you rise up with straightened legs, keep your heels raised and together.

- Inhale through your nose, move your buttocks back down to your heels and bring your head up so you are back in your starting position. Keep your fingertips on the floor for support.

- Going up and down like this is one complete round of Frog Pose.

- Be sure to keep connecting the breath with the movement, inhaling while lifting your head up and bringing your buttocks down to your lifted heels. Exhale, straightening your legs and bowing your head.

- Repeat for up to 10 rounds if this is your first time and gradually build up to 54 rounds.

- When you have finished, come to a seated position and stretch your legs forward. Take a few slower breaths to close the practice.

- Your muscles may be sore the next day, but this is a great indication you have had a good workout without needing to go to the gym.

Tip: No matter how many rounds you can manage, going slowly doesn't make it easier! It can actually make it feel harder, so see if you can pick up a brisk pace.

BREATHING UP (1:2)

Like accumulating interest on your bank account, starting small and practising this powerful exercise regularly can provide exponential benefits to your body, mind and overall wellbeing.

It is called "breathing up" because it is a technique taught in free-dive schools to help divers relax before holding their breath during dives. The long exhale induces a state of relaxation via parasympathetic stimulation and reducing surplus carbon dioxide levels in the body, which is one of the secrets to holding your breath for longer.

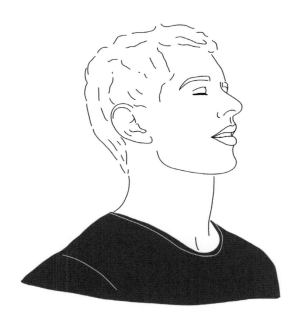

b e n e f i t s

Builds strength

Builds stamina

Balances nervous system

Stimulates red blood cell production

○ Sit or lie down in a comfortable position.

○ Breathe in (through the nose) using the diaphragm fully for a slow count of 5.

○ Then release the breath with a "Sssssss" sound like the air coming out of a tyre for slow count of 10.

○ Hold the breath for a moment at the end of the exhale.

○ Repeat 5 times.

With practice, you can begin to increase the length of the inhalation and exhalation but stick with the same 1:2 ratio. You can build up to a practice of 20–30 rounds.

DID YOU KNOW?

Consistent practice of healthy breath-holding has been shown to increase erythropoietin (EPO) production in kidneys, the hormone which triggers red blood cell production. It's like high-altitude training in the privacy of your own home!

REFERENCES

A Life Worth Breathing by Max Strom
The Oxygen Advantage by Patrick McKeown
Perfect Breathing by Al Lee and Don Campbell
Principals of Anatomy and Physiology by Gerard J. Tortora and Bryan H. Derrickson
The Breathing Book by Donna Fahri

www.alchemyofbreath.com
www.beencaughthealing.com
www.claritybreathwork.com
www.inspirationalbreathing.com
www.mumsforlungs.com
www.omocado.com
www.quotegarden.com
https://www.researchgate.net/profile/Federico_Brilli
www.schoolbreathe.com
www.stressresolutionformen.com
www.sybille.com
www.thebreathingroom.co.uk
www.transformationalbreath.co.uk
www.stancortes.com

Thank Yous

They say it takes a village to raise a child, and I can safely say it takes a city to write a book! From this books early life, a huge thank you to Lauren Gardner of Bell Lomax Moreton, who guided me throughout. Thank you to Vicky Orchard, editor, from Kyle Books for your vision, style and all round brilliance. To Mira Lou Kellner...thank YOU for breathing a breath of life into every page with your beautiful illustrations and boundless talent. Thank you to Joanna Copestick, for giving me the amazing opportunity to write and publish a book. To Nikki Dupin, Emma Wells and Abby Cocovini of Studio nic and lou – thank you for your brilliant design work and Lisa Pinnell, and everyone at Kyle Books for producing such a handsome tome! Thank you to Mauricio Corridan of Omocado for your generosity of spirit and allowing us to use your photography as the source of inspiration for some of the illustrations in this book.

Massive thanks to everyone who agreed to offer their expertise and advice to share amongst these pages. To all who appear in the book and to all those behind the scenes: Mel Lacy Fewtrell aka @breathgal you are a legend! To Sig Watkins of Fit MG, John Collins, Rob De, Dr Ben Marshall, Frederico Brilli, huge thanks for answering all my questions!

To those who are a constant source of love and laughter. I'm lucky to be supported in all four directions: To the North, my best friend ever, Livesey, Audrey would be proud! Big love to Sarah Anderson, for your kind heart and belief in the School Breathe project.

To the West – Thank you to Nick for putting up with me tapping away on a laptop for near on eternity. Massive hugs to you, and the entire Cunard Family, for your love and support. Big cheers to Charlie Davey for being a constant source of humour, Tash Gothard, for your friendship and for being the calmest person I know. I'm still learning from you! Grazie Mille to Adrian and Corinne of Evolve Wellness Centre for all your support and inspiration.

To the South, Kate Peers, aka Longers, for all your nudges of encouragement and for being a brilliant friend.

To the East – Abby McLachlan & East of Eden THANK YOU for all the opportunities you have offered me over the last few years. To Hannah Goodman for being a magical part of the School Breathe vision. Thank you to James Green, Headmaster at Sebright, for embracing breathwork with such enthusiasm. To my clients, who are a constant source of inspiration. To all those in the breathwork community who have offered their time and support to help facilitate my workshops, events and retreats. To the E17 mums and dads who have unknowingly kept me sane. To Jasmin, for all the last-minute childcare requests and your pockets of wisdom.

To the South West - my home, my heart. To Mum, for your dedicated read-throughs, "advice", teas on tap, and uplifting support. To Dad, for always bringing humour into my life and a HUGE cheers to you both for looking after Rabs and Dolly, so I could complete the task in hand. You are the best grandparents and I love you so much. To Sam and Ben for being the best trouts in the world. Love you!

Lastly, to the most influential teachers in love and life, my inhale and my exhale and all of those in between, Hartley and Ava, thank you for giving me the best job on earth, love and magic always – your mum xx